Providing Home Care for Older Adults

A practical guide to providing home-based mental health services, *Providing Home Care for Older Adults* teaches readers how to handle the unique aspects of home-based care and apply and adapt evidence-based assessment and treatment within the home-based setting.

Featuring contributions from experienced, board-certified home care psychologists, social workers, and psychiatrists, the book explains the multifaceted role of a home-based provider, offers concrete and practical considerations for working within the home, and highlights adaptations to specific evidence-based methods used in treating homebound older adults. Also covered are special topics related to hoarding, safety, capacity evaluations, caregivers, case management, and use of technology. Each chapter includes engaging case examples with practical tips that illustrate what it is like to work in this new and exciting frontier.

Psychologists, counselors, and other mental health practitioners in home settings will be able to use this guide to provide effective home-based care to older adults.

Danielle L. Terry, PhD, ABPP, is a board-certified health psychologist and Director of Behavioral Science at the Guthrie Medical Center Family Medicine Residency in Sayre, Pennsylvania.

Michelle E. Mlinac, PsyD, ABPP, is a board-certified geropsychologist at VA Boston Healthcare System who has worked in home-based primary care since 2008. She is an assistant professor of psychology in the Department of Psychiatry at Harvard Medical School, Boston, Massachusetts.

Pamela L. Steadman-Wood, PhD, ABPP, is a board-certified geropsychologist. She has worked for the Providence VA Medical Center's home-based primary care program since 2007. She is also an associate professor in the Department of Psychiatry and Human Behavior at the Warren Alpert Medical School of Brown University, Providence, Rhode Island.

Providing Home Care for Older Adults

A Professional Guide for Mental Health Practitioners

Edited by Danielle L. Terry, Michelle E. Mlinac, and Pamela L. Steadman-Wood

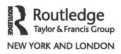

Routledge
Taylor & Francis Group

NEW YORK AND LONDON

First published 2021
by Routledge
52 Vanderbilt Avenue, New York, NY 10017

and by Routledge
2 Park Square, Milton Park, Abingdon, Oxon, OX14 4RN

Routledge is an imprint of the Taylor & Francis Group, an informa business

© 2021 Taylor & Francis

The right of Danielle L. Terry, Michelle E. Mlinac, and Pamela
L. Steadman-Wood to be identified as the authors of the editorial
material, and of the authors for their individual chapters, has been
asserted in accordance with sections 77 and 78 of the Copyright, Designs
and Patents Act 1988.

Library of Congress Cataloging-in-Publication Data
Names: Terry, Danielle L., editor. | Mlinac, Michelle E., editor. |
Steadman-Wood, Pamela L., editor.
Title: Providing home care for older adults : a professional
guide for mental health practitioners / edited by, Danielle
L. Terry, Michelle E. Mlinac, Pamela L. Steadman-Wood.
Identifiers: LCCN 2020013029 (print) | LCCN 2020013030 (ebook) |
ISBN 9780367345266 (hardback) | ISBN 9780367345273 (paperback) |
ISBN 9780429326363 (ebook)
Subjects: MESH: Home Care Services | Mental Health Services |
Health Services for the Aged | Mental Disorders–therapy | Mental
Disorders–diagnosis | Veterans Health Services | Aged
Classification: LCC RA645.3 (print) | LCC RA645.3 (ebook) |
NLM WT 31 | DDC 362.2/4–dc23
LC record available at https://lccn.loc.gov/2020013029
LC ebook record available at https://lccn.loc.gov/2020013030

ISBN: 978-0-367-34526-6 (hbk)
ISBN: 978-0-367-34527-3 (pbk)
ISBN: 978-0-429-32636-3 (ebk)

Typeset in Times
by Swales & Willis, Exeter, Devon, UK

This book is dedicated to those that we are privileged to serve in home care. And to Mrs. S., who once said, "Are you the maid who keeps my secrets?"

Contents

Contributors

Ami Bryant, PhD, is a clinical psychologist who specializes in working with older adults and rural populations. She has worked for the Puget Sound VA Medical Center Home-Based Primary Care (HBPC) Program on the Olympic Peninsula since 2016. Her research interests include health disparities among older adults as well as substance use and abuse among older adults.

Tamarra Crawford, PhD, ABPP, is a board-certified specialist in geropsychology. She has worked as a psychologist in HBPC and in the skilled nursing Community Living Center of VA hospitals for 13 years. Her interests include developmental milestones, interdisciplinary team functioning, diversity, and geropsychology.

Courtney O. Ghormley, PhD, ABPP, is a board-certified specialist in geropsychology. She has worked at the Central Arkansas Veterans Healthcare System for the past 10 years and serves as a geropsychologist in the HBPC program. She also serves as Director of Training for the psychology internship program. Her clinical interests include cognitive assessment, the diagnosis and management of dementia, and caregiver education and support.

William Gibson, PhD, is a clinical psychologist and neuropsychologist who has worked in the VA system for over 13 years, almost six of those in home care. His interests include working with various responses to trauma (PTSD, moral injury, and traumatic grief and loss), working with older adults, and working people at the end of life. He is currently the Program Coordinator for the residential PTSD programs at the Batavia (NY) VA.

Megan E. Gomez, PhD, is a clinical psychologist working at the Tibor Rubin Medical Center, VA Long Beach Healthcare System, in the HBPC program. She provides clinical psychology services to Veterans enrolled in the program and their caregivers and facilitates the Parkinson's Support Group at VA Long Beach. Her research interests include cognitive health in older adults and improving the quality of life for people with Parkinson's disease.

Harriette Grooh, PhD, CMC, a licensed clinical psychologist and certified care manager, has worked in geropsychology for nearly 40 years. She is the founder of HGA Personal Care Consultants, a private interdisciplinary consultation and care management firm in the San Francisco Bay Area. She created the first mobile geriatric evaluation team for Marin County Community Health Services before starting HGA. She is one of the founding directors of the Alzheimer's Association of Northern California and Northern Nevada and served on the Board of Directors of the Aging Life Care Association (ALCA), formerly known as the National Association of Professional Geriatric Care Managers, and is one of the founding directors and past president of the 12-state Western Region Chapter of ALCA. She is a board director of the National Academy of Certified Care Managers.

Kimberly E. Hiroto, PhD, is a clinical geropsychologist at the Palo Alto VA Health Care System. She previously worked in HBPC at another VA prior to her current position in Hospice and Palliative Care. She has served on various workgroups and committees within the American Psychological Association's Office on Aging, focused on advocating for older adults' mental health, and continues serving on local and national committees focused on aging, social justice, and multicultural diversity. Her professional interests include interdisciplinary education and training in geropsychology, palliative care, and diversity.

Carolyn T. Jackson, PhD, is a clinical psychologist who has worked for the Syracuse VA Medical Center's HBPC program for 10 years. Dr. Jackson is also a Veteran whose research interests include the relationship between military cultural experience and clinical issues among Veterans, as well as the delivery of empirically-supported clinical interventions to those who reside in rural and/or socioeconomically disadvantaged communities.

Ann T. Landes, PhD, is a staff psychologist at the Syracuse VA Medical Center. Trained at the San Antonio VA in geropsychology and palliative care, Dr. Landes has worked in diverse settings within medical centers and outpatient clinics during her tenure of 15-plus years with the Department of Veterans Affairs. Her areas of expertise include: health psychology, aging across the lifespan, adjustment to disability, end-of-life issues, and family systems.

Angela W. Lau, PhD, is a staff psychologist for the HBPC Program at the Tibor Rubin Medical Center, VA Long Beach Healthcare System. She has provided home-based psychological services to Veterans and their family caregivers for over 11 years. Her areas of professional interest and clinical specialization include clinical geropsychology, behavioral medicine, anxiety disorders, and minority mental health.

James "Chip" Long, PhD, ABPP, is a board-certified specialist in geropsychology. He has worked in an HBPC setting for 12 years, both at the Central Arkansas VA Medical Center and in the Veterans Healthcare System of the Ozarks. His clinical interests include the identification and treatment of psychological issues in the elderly and medically ill, assessment and monitoring of cognitive status in medical settings, and family caregiver support.

Michelle E. Mlinac, PsyD, ABPP, is a board-certified geropsychologist at VA Boston Healthcare System who has worked in HBPC since 2008. She is an assistant professor of psychology in the Department of Psychiatry at Harvard Medical School. Her research and clinical interests include problem-solving therapy, decision-making capacity, and geropsychology training. She serves on the Executive Committee of the American Board of Geropsychology (ABGERO), and is Chair-Elect of the Council of Professional Geropsychology Training Programs.

Marc Nespoli, MD, is a board-certified physician in geriatric psychiatry. Dr. Nespoli worked in the HBPC Program at VA Connecticut for seven years, before being recently appointed as the Medical Director for the Mental Health Clinic of the Newington campus. As an assistant clinical professor at Yale University, Dr. Nespoli has enjoyed taking residents and fellows on home visits in order to provide them with a unique learning experience.

Marc Parker, PsyD, is a psychology resident with Senior Connections in Vancouver, WA, where he provides psychological services to residents in long-term nursing care. He completed his predoctoral internship with Heritage Clinic in Pasadena, CA, and he attended Pacific University's School of Graduate Psychology in Hillsboro, OR. His research interests include the development of group psychotherapy interventions that address the unique needs of older adults.

Fred Pasche, LICSW, is a licensed independent clinical social worker who has worked in state government and public affairs. For the past 12 years he has focused on elder care issues as an inpatient case manager at VA Boston Healthcare System and more recently as a social worker with the HBPC team.

Donna Reulbach, LICSW, is a licensed independent clinical social worker who has worked in the field of elder care for 20 years. For the past eight years, she has served as a social worker in the HBPC team at VA Boston Healthcare System. Additionally, she has past experience doing home visits in the field of child welfare.

Luis Richter, PsyD, ABPP, is a board-certified specialist in health psychology. He has worked for the Puget Sound VA Medical Center HBPC Program in Seattle for five years. He also serves on the American Board of Clinical Health Psychology. His research interests include integrative medicine, weight management, and end-of-life care.

Rachel L. Rodriguez, PhD, ABPP, is a board-certified clinical geropsychologist. She has worked with the VA's HBPC Program since 2007, first at the VA Palo Alto Health Care System and currently at the VA Durham Health Care System. Her research interests include adjustment to chronic and life-limiting illness, geropsychology education and training, and workforce development programs to enhance access for geriatric mental health care.

Clair Rummel, PhD, ABPP, is a board-certified specialist in geropsychology. She has provided mental health care to older Veterans in both outpatient and home care settings since 2011. Her research interests include increasing access to care for older adults via telehealth and adjustment to disability.

Carlos Santell, PsyD, obtained his doctorate degree in Clinical Psychology from Carlos Albizu University, San Juan Campus. He has a graduate certificate in Gerontology from University of Puerto Rico. He completed his doctoral internship at Heritage Clinic, a community mental health agency serving adults and older adults. Dr. Santell is currently completing a post-doctoral position at Heritage Clinic, Los Angeles Office.

Shannon Sisco, PhD, is a clinical psychologist at the VA Illiana Healthcare System, where she has provided behavioral health services as an interdisciplinary team member in HBPC for three years. She also serves as a VA subject-matter expert in Problem Solving Training for Primary Care. She provides supervision to psychology trainees and training in clinical supervision to psychology staff. Her research interests include social determinants of health in aging.

Pamela L. Steadman-Wood, PhD, ABPP, is a board-certified clinical geropsychologist. She has worked for the Providence VA Medical Center's HBPC program for 12 years. She is also an associate professor in the Department of Psychiatry and Human Behavior at the Alpert Medical School of Brown University. Her research interests include integrated health care for older adults, geropsychology education and training, and evidence-based psychotherapy competency training.

Amanda R. W. Steiner, PhD, is a clinical psychologist at the VA San Diego Healthcare System where she has worked as a team member of the HBPC program for nine years. She is also affiliated with the Department of Psychiatry at the University of California, San Diego as an assistant clinical professor. She provides supervision to psychology trainees and is involved in teaching medical students. Her research interests include emotional functioning and well-being in older adulthood.

Maureen E. Sweeney, PsyD, is a licensed psychologist with a certificate in Post-Doctoral Geriatric Psychology Training from the New Jersey Institute for Successful Aging at Rowan University in Stratford, NJ. She operates a specialized geropsychology practice in Bensalem, PA. She has continued to develop, implement, and grow a private-practice model of delivering mental health services to older adults at home over the past 15 years.

Danielle L. Terry, PhD, ABPP, is a board-certified health psychologist and Director of Behavioral Science at the Guthrie Medical Center Family Medicine Residency in Sayre, PA. She worked in HBPC for five years. Her research interests include various topics in health psychology and residency training and education.

Julie Loebach Wetherell, PhD, ABPP, is a board-certified geropsychologist at the VA San Diego Healthcare System, where she directs behavioral medicine services as a member of the HBPC team, and Professor of Psychiatry at the University of California, San Diego, where she conducts research on geriatric mental health and teaches and supervises psychology and psychiatry trainees in research and clinical work. She is a past winner of the American Psychological Association Division 12 David Shakow Early Career Award and a Fellow of the Behavioral and Social Sciences Section of the Gerontological Society of America.

Janet Yang, PhD, ABPP, is a licensed and board-certified clinical geropsychologist with over 35 years' experience working with older adults. She is the Clinical Director and the Training Director at Heritage Clinic, a mental health and adult day care center serving older adults in Los Angeles, and trains graduate students in mental health fields. She has published articles and conducted training on psychotherapy with older adults, mental health outreach, reminiscence, and a variety of other topics related to mental health and aging.

Jenny Yen, PsyD, is an early-career geropsychologist. She completed a geropsychology post-doctoral fellowship at the VA Palo Alto Health Care System. Currently, she is the Training Director at the Institute on Aging. She provides consultation, as well as conducting assessment and behavioral health training for San Francisco and San Mateo counties. Her interests are dementia, capacity evaluations, sexuality, and advocating for underserved groups.

Brian Zuzelo, PhD, has worked as a psychologist in Bedford, MA at the Edith Nourse Rogers Memorial VA Hospital's HBPC program for the past 12 years. He developed and currently serves as the Administrator of the hospital's Geropsychology Outpatient Clinic. Dr. Zuzelo also collaborated in the design of the hospital's geropsychology training program, and where he continues to supervise doctoral-level trainees.

Foreword

It is an honor and a pleasure to help introduce this important book. As we all grapple with the enormous challenge of caring for an aging population with significant long-term care needs (e.g., Lynn, 2019), home-based care is a critical part of the continuum of health and personal care. While you might associate home-based medical care with the old-time country doctor making house calls, home-based primary care (HBPC) is a growing care model. In the United States, it is being widely implemented via both Medicare and the Department of Veterans Affairs (VA) health care systems (De Jonge et al., 2014; Edes et al., 2014; Leff et al., 2015; Schuchman, Fain, & Cornwell, 2018). And, of course, home-based nursing, rehabilitation, personal, and hospice care are important services that support older adults in recovering from a health setback, maintain functioning, and/or die in their homes. It is only quite recently that mental health professionals have been providing services in home settings, particularly in VA (Gillespie et al., 2019; Hicken & Plowhead, 2010; Karlin & Karel, 2014).

Older adults with multiple chronic conditions and, commonly, comorbid behavioral and mental health concerns often have difficulty accessing clinic-based care, including mental health services. Untreated mental illness – including depression, anxiety, substance use disorders, posttraumatic stress disorder, behavioral symptoms in dementia, and severe mental illness – is related to increased morbidity, functional disability, and mortality among older adults. If we are to improve access to mental health services for older adults with significant and complex comorbidities, mental health professionals need to consider providing care in the home – via home visits, telehealth care, and/or supporting teams that provide in-home care.

On a personal note, I've unfortunately had little personal experience providing mental health care in the home. Much of my career was spent working in an outpatient geriatric mental health clinic at a VA medical center, where I worked with older Veterans in individual, group, and family therapy contexts. I think back to how many times I really thought

I was getting to know someone until a family member, care manager, adult protective service worker, or other person who knew the Veteran and his/her home environment shared information that I simply wasn't aware of (e.g., the extent of hoarding, dilapidated or otherwise unsafe conditions, stockpiled medications). Likewise, over time I had a chance to do some home-based research interviews and to accompany VA HBPC psychologists on home visits. Seeing how someone functions in their everyday environment provides such a critical context for assessment and treatment that is difficult to replicate via interview in an office-based setting.

My career transitioned to an administrative one, in which I currently work for the Office of Mental Health and Suicide Prevention in the Department of Veterans Affairs Central Office (CO), serving as National Mental Health Director, Geriatric Mental Health. When I first went to work for VACO, I served as the Program Coordinator for the HBPC Mental Health Initiative; starting in 2007–2008, psychologists and/or psychiatrists began to be integrated into every VA HBPC program nationally per VA policy. Providing care in Veterans' homes, in collaboration with an interdisciplinary team, was certainly a new model of care for most of the people initially taking these jobs (and those who continue to fill them). We have worked to develop a model of integrated mental health care, and provide clinical, administrative, and training resources. If only we had the material now covered in this book to help orient staff to mental health care in the home!

It is so inspiring to hear stories about how mental health professionals are making a difference for Veterans, family caregivers, and teams in HBPC, as well as the joys and difficulties of the work, which challenge all notions of usual professional boundaries. Examples shared during one particularly heartfelt and sometimes hilarious email listserv discussion include: lifting a turkey out of the oven because the Veteran and his wife are too frail to get it out; arriving to find a patient on the floor or otherwise in the midst of a medical emergency; shoveling snow to get in the driveway/door; dealing with all sorts of pets, friendly and not, as well as farm and wild animals in rural and frontier areas; confronting bed bugs and an infinite variety of messy situations; changing light bulbs and teaching how to use a TV remote, cable, microwave; connecting with spouses, adult children, grandchildren, neighbors in all manner of interaction; dealing with flat tires or other car problems; setting off home security alarms; watching a couple in their nineties wink and gaze at each other as if newlyweds; finding how behavioral activation can mean observing and learning how to make borscht, baklava, black-eyed peas, and much, much more.

One person summarized the discussion very well: "I've got to say that I firmly believe that those of us who do home-based work have to be at the very top of our game in order to provide compassionate assessment and therapy services to our very vulnerable patients in very challenging environments! Makes me proud to do this kind of work with such amazing colleagues." Another person added, "There is no other Psychology job in the VA where you have to be culturally competent to the fullest. We understand urban/suburban/rural cultures. We learn about our patients based on their family, ethnic, racial, etc., cultures to work better with them because we're (literally) in the thick of it." And, "This is the best job and I couldn't imagine doing anything else. I get to stretch myself in new ways every day and have the opportunity to work with the most amazing patients and providers."

Of note, it has been nearly impossible to evaluate the clinical and cost impact of integrating mental health professionals in HBPC, given nationwide implementation and no reasonable comparison/control group. However, there is little doubt that access to mental health services is improving for these Veterans and that, based on team feedback and many anecdotes, HBPC mental health professionals are making a difference in contributing to holistic, biopsychosocial care in HBPC (Karlin & Karel, 2014).

This book is a gift for mental health professionals who would like to consider adding home-based work to their practice. The editors and authors are experienced clinicians with many years of experience providing home-based mental health care for older adults. The book addresses the ethical, clinical, practical, logistical, billing, personal, and interpersonal aspects of providing geriatric mental health services in the home. Case examples throughout give a flavor for this meaningful work, the variety of clinical issues and home environments, and how mental health professionals can make a difference for the well-being and quality of life of older adults, and their caregivers, who are doing the best they can to manage health and functional challenges in late life.

Michele J. Karel, Ph.D., ABPP
Board-Certified in Geropsychology
National Mental Health Director, Geriatric Mental Health
Office of Mental Health and Suicide Prevention
Department of Veterans Affairs Central Office

References

De Jonge, K. E., Jamshed, N., Gilden, D., Kubisiak, J., Bruce, S. R., & Taler, G. (2014). Effects of home-based primary care on Medicare costs in high-risk elders. *Journal of the American Geriatrics Society, 62*, 1825–1831. doi:10.1111/jgs.12974.

Edes, T., Kinosian, B., Vuckovic, N. H., Nichols, L. O., Becker, M. M., & Hossain, M. (2014). Better access, quality, and cost for clinically complex veterans with home-based primary care. *Journal of the American Geriatrics Society, 62*, 1954–1961. doi:10.1111/jgs.13030.

Gillespie, S. M., Manheim, C., Gilman, C., Karuza, J., Olsan, T. H., Edwards, S. T., ... Haverhals, L. (2019). Interdisciplinary team perspectives on mental health care in VA home-based primary care: A qualitative study. *American Journal of Geriatric Psychiatry, 27*, 128–137. doi:10.1016/j.jagp.2018.10.006.

Hicken, B. L., & Plowhead, A. (2010). A model for home-based psychology from the Veterans Health Administration. *Professional Psychology: Research and Practice, 41*, 340–346. doi:10.1037/a0020431.

Karlin, B. E., & Karel, M. L. (2014). National integration of MH practitioners in VA home-based primary care: An innovative model for mental health care delivery with older adults. *The Gerontologist, 54*(5), 868–879. doi:10.1093/geront/gnt142.

Leff, B., Weston, C. M., Garrigues, S., Patel, K., & Ritchie, C., for the National Home-Based Primary Care and Palliative Network. (2015). Home-based primary care practices in the United States: Current state and quality improvement approaches. *Journal of the American Geriatrics Society, 63*, 963–969. doi:10.1111/jgs.13382.

Lynn, J. (2019). The "fierce urgency of now": Geriatrics professionals speaking up for older adult care in the United States. *Journal of the American Geriatrics Society, 67*, 2001–2003. doi:10.1111/jgs.16116.

Schuchman, M., Fain, M., & Cornwell, T. (2018). The resurgence of home-based primary care models in the United States. *Geriatrics, 3*, 41. doi:10.3390/geriatrics3030041.

Part 1
What Is Home Care?

1 Introduction to Home-Based Mental Health Care

Models, Roles, and Reflections

Tamarra Crawford, Michelle E. Mlinac, Pamela L. Steadman-Wood, and Danielle L. Terry

Dr. Judy Chan, a psychologist who works as part of home care team, drives down a gravel road in the country to meet a new patient, Mr. Brown. His home care nurse hoped Dr. Chan could help Mr. Brown, an 83-year-old recently widowed man with chronic post-traumatic stress disorder (PTSD) and advancing Parkinson's disease, better follow his treatment plan. The visit was challenging at first. Mr. Brown was reluctant to answer questions, and told Dr. Chan that having doctors in his home made him nervous. Dr. Chan asked Mr. Brown what brought him joy despite his many health problems and recent loss of his husband. Mr. Brown shared that his beloved horses depended on him for care. Dr. Chan asked for a tour of the barn and to meet the horses, and Mr. Brown smiled with relief and escorted her to the stables. They agreed that whenever possible, future home care visits would be held in there, where Mr. Brown felt most comfortable. During their first psychotherapy visits together, Mr. Brown taught Dr. Chan how to feed, water, and brush the horses. As the therapy relationship developed, Mr. Brown opened about his frustrations with his limitations and fear that if he declined further (physically or mentally) he would be unable to care for his horses. Dr. Chan helped Mr. Brown focus on his value of taking care of his horses and appreciate that accepting assistance and taking his medications as prescribed would help him stay strong enough to do so. With increased trust, Mr. Brown was willing to meet with other members of the team, and over time agreed to engage in evidence-based treatment to better address his PTSD symptoms. With symptom improvement, Mr. Brown eventually agreed to have home health aides assist him in better caring for himself. His medical and psychiatric symptoms stabilized, and Mr. Brown was able to spend several months caring for his horses independently. When unable to care for them alone, he hired help to do so. With the trust of the home care team, Mr. Brown was able to identify his end-of-life wishes and treatment preferences. When the time came, he accepted a referral to home hospice. With their support, he was able to spend his last days in a hospital bed in the sunroom of his home overlooking the barn, when he took his last breath, peacefully and with dignity.

This case illustrates the value of a home care service that includes an integrated mental health (MH) provider who can address the unique needs of older adult patients. Individuals receiving home care often have complex health and behavioral health care needs, including advanced illness, comorbid psychiatric conditions, and complex psychosocial issues. They may be high utilizers of the health care system, having frequent hospitalizations, emergency room visits, and rehabilitation stays. Care delivered in the home seeks to address these complexities, to improve access to MH treatment, to align delivered care with the patient's personal goals, and to reduce unneeded or overly burdensome healthcare.

MH providers, including psychologists, psychiatrists, psychiatric nurse practitioners and nurses, counselors, and clinical social workers, have a vital role to play in meeting the MH care needs for this population of older adults. This book is the first to describe this evolving model of geriatric MH practice within the patient's home. The aims of this book are: to spark the reader's interest in this type of clinical work, to describe practical strategies for assessment and treatment, and to highlight the powerful impact that can be made when patients are met in their homes. While home-based care can be challenging, it is counterbalanced by the privilege of being invited into the homes of patients and their families, by the joys of working with an engaged interdisciplinary team or flying solo as a provider, and by the successes of resources to help older adults meet their goals of aging-in-place. This book is written primarily by experienced home care psychologists, with contributions from psychiatry and social work providers. Each chapter includes case examples and practical tips that illustrate what it is like to work in this new frontier of MH care. We invited authors with expertise and passion for this type of work to contribute to this book, with the hope it will engage future practitioners in home care.

Overview of the Book

This book is divided into three main sections. Part 1 focuses on the foundational and practical aspects of home-based MH care. Later in this chapter, we review models of home care for older adults, and identify the many roles and skills the MH provider brings to the job. Chapter 2 further explores the home care MH provider's role within the healthcare team. Chapter 3 describes the process of developing a therapeutic relationship when providing home-based MH care, with important ethical and cultural considerations in treatment. Part 2 focuses on the practical aspects of home care. Chapter 4 explores how working out of each patient's home and using a mobile office differ from traditional clinic-based work. In Chapter 5, a psychologist shares her experiences of developing her own home-based MH private practice, an innovative model that could be replicated by other providers interested in this type of work. Safety issues in providing home care, including driving hazards, infection control, and home oxygen, are reviewed in Chapter 6, with recommendations on how to be prepared for unexpected situations. Hoarding is a common concern in home care, and a brief review of assessment and intervention strategies are found in Chapter 7. Unique considerations for social workers and psychiatry providers who provide home care are explored in chapters 8 and 9 respectively. Part 3 covers assessment and interventions in the home. Logistics of providing home-based psychodiagnostic and cognitive evaluations in the home are illustrated in Chapter 10. Many patients in home care require evaluations of decision-making capacity for issues related to health care, independent living, and financial management, as reviewed in Chapter 11. Chapter 12 gives consideration to evidence-based psychotherapy delivered in the home. Chapter 13 provides a guide to caregiver interventions that are critical in supporting the home care patient's family and friends who serve in these stressful roles. Home care provides an important learning environment for MH trainees, and Chapter 14 describes the roles of the MH practitioner in educating both trainees and the team. Finally, Chapter 15 explores emerging areas in home care: suicide prevention, behavioral medicine interventions, telehealth, and end-of-life care.

Home-Delivered Healthcare in the Twenty-First Century

House calls, once commonplace, were on the decline for much of the twentieth century. Over the past several decades, home care for older adults has been making a comeback. Reasons for the revival of this model in the United States include increased demand for home-based service provision, health care reform, and the evidence demonstrating the benefits of home-based care (Schuchman, Fain, & Cornwell, 2018). Older adults are the most rapidly growing sector of the population as people are living longer and preferring to age-in-place. The subset of older adults served by home-based health care programs such as home-based primary care (HBPC) or home hospice are generally those whose complex health issues are not well-met by more traditional outpatient care. The incidence of chronic medical conditions increases with age and contributes to functional impairment that makes it difficult to access outpatient care. These health and functional challenges can increase the risk of psychiatric disorders such as depression and anxiety. Access to MH care treatment for older adults with complex medical conditions and functional limitations is limited (Borson et al., 2019). These access issues lead to missed appointments, fragmented care, and sub-optimally controlled medical conditions. Poor access to care leads to increased health care utilization (e.g., emergency room visits, extended hospital lengths of stay and nursing home placement etc.), which is costly. Integrated home-based care helps improve access to medical and MH care, reduce health care utilization, and delay nursing home placement (Schuchman, Fain, & Cornwell, 2018).

Models of Home Care

Home care models come in all shapes and sizes but can be categorized as government-funded (Medicare, Department of Veterans Affairs), hospital-based or academic-affiliated, and free-standing programs. HBPC provides patient-centered, comprehensive, longitudinal care in the homes of patients with complex medical, psychiatric, and functional-related conditions not managed effectively by routine outpatient care. All HBPC programs differ on the mission, payment structure, and role within the health system. In contrast to the services provided by visiting nurse agencies (which are typically short-term and problem-focused), HBPC teams aim to foster a long-term patient care relationship that incorporates end-stage disease care management, caregiver support, and emerging technologies like telehealth.

The Veterans Administration (later the Department of Veterans Affairs, or VA) developed one of the first HBPC services in 1972 to address the increasing population of Veterans with chronic complex illness and associated functional impairment (Beales & Edes, 2009; Karlin & Karel, 2014). Off-shoots of the VA model have been implemented by Medicare to address the needs of individuals recently discharged from a hospital admission to reduce the risk of readmission, and provision of care to individuals living in assisted-living facilities and group homes. Hospital-based programs have implemented HBPC programs targeting patients with the most complex and costliest conditions (Mount Sinai Visiting Doctors Program, or MSVDP; Reckrey et al., 2014). Many of these home-based programs started out with a focus on stabilizing chronic medical conditions. More recently, home care programs like VA HBPC and MSVDP have recognized the need for addressing the psychosocial needs of patients served by home care services, including Independence-at-Home (Center for Medicare Services' HBPC demonstration program). As such, programs integrating mental and behavioral health services have been shown to be efficacious in improving access to medical and MH care, reducing health care utilization, and delaying nursing home placement.

Home-based care is a dynamic system of services, needs, and interprofessional work. Hospitals and medical systems, such as the VA, integrate MH practitioners (psychologists and psychiatrists) and social workers within home-visiting primary care and geriatric teams made up of physicians, registered nurses, nurse practitioners, physician assistants, dieticians, rehabilitation therapists, and pharmacists. MH home care may be provided within an interdisciplinary medical or primary care team. For other organizations or community agencies, care is provided as an adjunctive service, or even as a stand-alone service (Reifler & Bruce, 2014). Home-based MH work may also be the focus or part of a private practice. As this evolving model of integrated health care emerges, it may also be new and surprising for patients, families, and fellow health care providers. This may require enthusiastic and frequent education about home-based MH care to others outside (and sometimes inside!) the MH field.

Home hospice (or home-based palliative care – an emerging model) may be more familiar to patients and their families, and the composition and general day-to-day functioning of the team may be similar. In these programs, social workers, chaplains, or psychologists may provide both direct in-home MH care to patients (and their loved ones) at the very end of life and offer bereavement support to grieving families after the patient dies. Home hospice and palliative care teams may be augmented with other types of complementary care, such as art or music therapy.

Roles of the Home-Based MH Provider

Diagnostician

Being a front-line service provider in the home requires wearing many hats. A primary responsibility is to conduct a comprehensive MH assessment, determine a psychiatric diagnosis, and offer clinical recommendations. Home-based MH providers must effectively translate psychodiagnostic information and recommendations so that they are jargon-free and may be understood and effectively implemented by patients, families, and team members. For example, the MH provider may advise the team how to teach the patient medical information in a way that they can understand, utilize written materials or caregiver supports, or make slow, simple changes to dietary or exercise behaviors.

Psychotherapist

An MH provider will naturally be aware of potential points of intervention for a variety of MH disorders. The challenge for the home-based provider is to assess how to deliver effective, evidence-based interventions in the context of intersecting medical, functional, and social complexities often unique to a home-based setting.

Team Member

Whether or not they are formally a part of a team, the MH provider will often collaborate and work closely with nurses, nurse practitioners, rehabilitation therapists, dieticians, physicians, pharmacists, or other providers to deliver effective care. Thus, MH providers should be able to engage in effective team communication, problem evaluation, and collaborative solution-finding.

Caregiver Support and Family Therapist

Training in family systems and group therapies can be helpful, as the home-based MH provider often intervenes with families and caregivers, providing psychoeducation, coaching in behavior management for dementia, assisting with communication dynamics, and identifying goals of care.

Care Manager

Often another team member (such as a nurse) may act as the primary manager of the patient's care, while the MH provider collaborates with the team around shared care management activities (appointment reminders, facilitating transportation, etc.). In some cases, in order for a community or legally based intervention to be successfully addressed, the MH provider may need to be the primary point of contact. For example, intensive care management may be required for someone presenting with severe self-neglect due to dementia (i.e. forgetting to eat, engaging in wandering, use of a stove or other burn/fire hazards) who is living alone without available caregivers. The MH provider may interface frequently with an adult protective services (APS) worker, or court-appointed guardian, to directly advocate for the patient's needs and develop a collaborative care plan.

Risk Manager

Due to the intimate nature of providing care in a patient's own home, there are a variety of unique situations MH providers may encounter. While such events are uncommon, MH providers should be prepared to handle high-risk, crisis, or reportable events. MH providers can ensure that neglect and abuse, or elevated-risk situations (e.g., suicidality) are evaluated; communicated to the team, patient, and family; and reported to the appropriate agencies as needed. Home care teams may ask all staff to be aware of protocols relating to infection control (e.g., handwashing, education, and provision of vaccinations), the posting and usage of home oxygen, falls prevention, or other home safety (e.g., fire alarms and clutter).

Educator

MH providers serve as expert trainers to their teams on all topics related to mental health. They foster competence in MH care management across their teams, as all interprofessional team members play a role in psychological wellness, prevention, and treatment of psychiatric issues. As home care is a rich interprofessional learning environment, the MH provider may supervise trainees to deliver effective care.

The Need for a Broad Knowledge and Training Base

Because the MH provider is often the front line of care, working alone in the field, being fluent in general MH practices is critical. Specialty training in areas such as geropsychology/geriatric psychiatry, health psychology, primary care, palliative care, and rehabilitation psychology are highly valuable additional skill sets.

Generalist Practices

MH providers in home care should have a versatile basic set of skills they bring into home visits, not limited to efficient rapport-building, flexibility, and patience, along with sharp psychodiagnostic, consultation, and intervention skills. They can expect a variety of common presenting problems such as anxiety, depression, and cognitive impairment as well as more complex medical and MH comorbidities, frequently compounded by loneliness and isolation. Familiarity with local policies and procedures, a strong foundation of ethical behavior, and a fluency with triaging complex cases are also key to a successful home care practice. With a strong foundation in generalist MH care, the following additional competencies are highly useful in this setting.

Geropsychology

In many respects, the practice of geropsychology was built for home-based care. While not all patients served by home care are older adults (for example, they may be young or middle-aged adults with early-onset dementia, movement disorders, or traumatic brain injury), by and large the population is over the age of 60. Geropsychology incorporates an understanding of lifespan development, geriatric care settings, collaborative interprofessional work, and normative aging, all of which are relevant to home-based care. A working knowledge of how MH issues can shift in presentation as a person ages can be key to promoting well-being and avoiding psychiatric decompensation. Within home care, it is important for the MH provider be attuned to the unique needs of older adults by selecting assessments and interventions appropriate for them, evaluating cultural and environmental factors, and working to combat age-related biases they encounter.

Health and Primary Care Psychology

Knowledge of health psychology will enhance the conceptualizations, treatments, and contributions of an MH provider within an interdisciplinary home-based team (American Psychological Association, 2008). Offering interventions such as smoking cessation, weight management, chronic pain management, help with adherence issues, or other behavioral medicine treatments will provide a dimension to care that can improve patient outcomes. In addition, it can be advantageous to understand mental health within a broader context, including how physical and mental health interface. When the MH provider is an integrated part of the healthcare team, they can improve access to care and reduce stigma for older adults, many whom may never have received MH treatment before. The MH provider may conduct joint visits with other members and receive "warm handoffs" to facilitate acceptance of care. MH providers who work as part of these teams can help the team identify, measure, and collaborate around treatment goals for each patient. In these ways, the MH provider may contribute to integrated preventative care, population health, or chronic disease management.

Rehabilitation Psychology

Having experience treating people with disabilities, working in acute rehabilitation settings, or helping injured or ill patients to recover functioning are all useful to inform MH practice in home care. While most patients wish to remain in their home as long as possible, that environment does not always match their needs. The interdisciplinary home care team typically addresses safety issues such as falls, swallowing problems, injury risks, or other hazards. The MH provider can address adaptation to loss, adherence to home rehabilitation, and comorbid MH and cognitive issues that can interfere with overall functioning.

Palliative Care and Hospice

Home-based MH providers can assist an interdisciplinary team or family caregiving system in implementing palliative care or hospice, including patient-driven care discussions, discussions of palliation alongside curative treatments, pain management, and recognizing when to revisit goals of care or engage in end-of-life planning when there are signs of imminent decline of health. MH providers can also assist with team dynamics when processing the reactions of health professionals, the patient, or family members and caregivers.

Identifying Your Role as a Home-Based MH Provider

Dr. Sora is a psychiatrist new to home care who has taken a position as the MH provider for a newly developed HBPC program. Prior to meeting with the HBPC team for the first time, Dr. Sora wonders about how to communicate his role and responsibilities to his team members, specific duties he might provide, and the frequency of his patient visits. During the meeting, Dr. Sora discovers other team members have differing experiences with MH providers and varying opinions about their value to the team. Quickly, Dr. Sora realizes that some team members want him to see as many patients as possible without them appreciating how to effectively triage and manage a complex patient panel. Realizing that he is unable to clearly articulate the answer himself, he is left asking himself the question, "How do I develop a strategy to triage my patients, and how do I explain to my team what I do?"

One of the primary challenges for MH providers is to understand and clarify what role and responsibilities they have individually and as a collective. Given that there are a variety of roles that one might have in home-care settings, how do MH providers know what role they might be functioning in at any given time? There are several factors to consider when determining what the next assessment, intervention, or case management steps might be.

Understand the Structure of Your Program

Understanding the infrastructure of the organization within which one works, and available resources, may dictate how one functions within the home. The structure and availability of resources of the work environment can vary significantly across teams. In addition, the MH provider must also understand the roles and responsibilities of their colleagues on the team. For example, the team's social worker may take the lead on family meetings and care coordination, while the team's psychologist may offer more intensive family therapy. Ideally, the MH provider is deployed judiciously. For example, older patients who can still drive to an outpatient visit to see their longtime psychiatrist do not necessarily need to receive home-based MH care just because they receive other home care services. Negotiating your role and responsibilities to a larger home care team will likely be an ongoing process.

Know the Culture of Your Program and the Population Served

Knowing the culture and traditions within a geographical area, a hospital system, or even a longstanding home care team can be beneficial to MH providers attempting to carve out their own roles. Over time, the addition of new members on a team may shift the team's culture.

Awareness of the history and culture of the geographical area being served is of benefit to the home-based MH provider visiting the home. While patients and families being treated in an outpatient setting may be prepared to share a more neutral space with items, structure, and medical approaches that indicate a culture that is new or different, those being visited in the home are surrounded by items, structure, and quite often family or neighbors which all serve to reinforce and maintain the cultural and traditional aspects of their life. Some patients and families may have strong values regarding how they accept persons into their home, regardless of intention or role. This can include offering and remaining in a formal space to meet versus the kitchen table or living area, offering food, requesting recognition of pets or other family members during the interaction, or even some participation in events coinciding with the visit (i.e. a family anniversary, birthday, or recognition of a family achievement).

There may be historical events that impact how mental health or other medical providers are perceived in a geographic region, especially within areas where medical care may have been limited for minority groups, or in geographical areas with strong recall of medical research or government programs that have adversely impacted one segment of the population over another. Dependent on location, there may also be a distant or recent history of social stratification. The patient or family may assume socio-ethnic or political status of the home-based visiting MH provider that may impact the therapeutic relationship. Having the awareness that this may occur, the ability to consult with diversity experts and/or community historians, and the rapport to gradually explore any interactions with family members, can greatly benefit the establishment of goals of care.

If a provider works within a larger medical system, it is important to be aware of how the MH, social work, and administrative bodies view the function of the home care team. It may also be helpful to reference one's organizational mission or goals when determining the provider's role. For example, the VA identified the primary goal of HBPC as preventing repeated hospitalizations while maintaining quality of life and safe independence at the maximum level of care and comfort. It can be beneficial to understand how each person on the team understands their own role within that complex goal.

Education and negotiation of roles, competencies, the nature of triage, resources, and time constraints are beneficial issues to target during introduction of a newly formed team or one undergoing restructuring. Consider requesting specific meetings with stakeholders to discuss their role and clarify their duties. Providing written materials or handouts to stakeholders about how to refer or triage can help others understand how you will function as a home-based provider.

Identify the Customer

In collaborative care models there are numerous stakeholders, including the patient, the family, professional caregivers, or other medical providers. Sometimes, the focus of evaluation and intervention lies entirely with the patient and is even solicited by the patient. Many times, the focus of education, collaboration, and change may not necessarily be with the patient, but with another stakeholder, or with the governing administration. For example, a nurse practitioner may want a family member to have better outcomes with feeding the patient a more nutritious diet to prevent weight loss. Although the intervention with the family involves the patient, the family, and the provider, the intervention and assessment provided is in service of the nurse practitioner's goals. In addition, although the intervention may directly benefit the patient's health according to typical medical guidelines, it may not align with the patient's actual goals or values, especially if the patient is in hospice care and does not want to eat due to discomfort. In this scenario, the "customer" is the medical provider.

Once the home-based provider has identified whom they are "working for," there may be a clear shift in the role that she or he is functioning within (e.g., evaluator, interventionist, educator). Aside from the patient, the provider may have referrals from APS, family members who have a desire to see the patient change in specific ways, caregivers or attorneys who request cognitive evaluations, or medical providers who have specific concerns about non-adherent behaviors.

The home-based MH provider will receive a variety of requests from stakeholders. In these instances, it is important to clarify the clinical question, and determine whose needs or goals are being addressed by the referral question. It is important to act in the best interest of the patient, and by identifying who the customer is, the provider can then determine their own roles and responsibilities.

When Roles Conflict

The act of providing care in another person's home may shift certain aspects of the traditional therapeutic framework. As such, boundaries and roles tend to be more flexible than in the outpatient setting. For example, home-based providers conduct care with patients who are in their pajamas, interact with beloved pets, meet lifelong best friends and new grandchildren of their patients, and enter the home during breakfast, lunch, and dinner. Given the numerous roles that providers may have, it is inevitable that those roles will occasionally conflict. Furthermore, providers will often be pulled to do things outside of their scope of practice for legitimate reasons.

Commonly Conflicting Roles

One of the most commonly conflicting roles in home-based care is that of an assessor and a therapist. Although it can be common in settings that serve adults of all ages to begin with a psychological intake, it is not as common to have to have the intake uncover concerns about abuse or neglect of an older person. In outpatient settings, evidence of abuse or neglect is identified by verbal report or obvious signs during clinic visits or hospitalizations. In home care, the population is arguably more vulnerable than a typical outpatient population, and observations from the home (rather than just subjective report) may result in a mandated report to APS. If working within a team, an MH provider may be confronted with outside information that the patient may not have normally shared (e.g., a severely dilapidated home or family members intimidating the patient during the visit, family members providing information the patient would not have volunteered). In these cases, being clear about the patient's decision-making capacity, status of durable powers of attorney or health care agent designations, reviewing ethics codes, consulting with teammates, or seeking guidance from a local ethics committee can be helpful to sort out what is in accordance with professional, ethical, and legal guidelines.

Summary

The home-based MH provider has numerous roles and responsibilities. Understanding the agency or organizational mission and regulations can guide the primary responsibilities that one may have. In addition to generalist training, developing skills in geropsychology, primary care, and health psychology can be valuable when providing care to a medically complex older adult population. With their strengths in communication, collaboration, and education, MH providers enhance the potential for positive outcomes for the patient, the family, and the interdisciplinary team.

References

American Psychological Association. (2008). *Blueprint for change: Achieving integrated health care for an aging population.* Retrieved from www.apa.org/pi/aging/programs/integrated/integrated-healthcare-report.pdf.

Beales, J.L., & Edes, T. (2009). Veteran's affairs home-based primary care. *Clinics in Geriatric Medicine, 25*(1), 149–154. doi:10.1016/j.cger.2008.11.002.

Borson, S., Korpak, A., Carbajal-Madrid, P., Likar, D., Brown, G.A., & Batra, R. (2019). Reducing barriers to mental health care: Bringing evidence-based psychotherapy home. *Journal of the American Geriatrics Society*, Advance online publication. doi:10.1111/jgs.10688.

Karlin, B.E., & Karel, M.L. (2014). National integration of MH practitioners in VA home-based primary care: An innovative model for mental health care delivery with older adults. *The Gerontologist*, *54*(5), 868–879. doi:10.1093/geront/gnt142.

Reckrey, J.M., Gettenberg, G.G., Ross, H., Kopke, V., Soriano, T., & Ornstein, K. (2014). The critical role of social workers in home-based primary care. *Social Work Health Care*, *53*(4), 330–343. doi:10.1080/00981389.2014.884041.

Reifler, B.V., & Bruce, M.L. (2014). Home-based mental health services for older adults: A review of ten model programs. *American Journal of Geriatric Psychiatry*, *22*, 241–247. doi:10.1016/j.jagp.2012.12.002.

Schuchman, M., Fain, M., & Cornwell, T. (2018). The resurgence of home-based primary care models in the United States. *Geriatrics*, *3*, 41. doi:10.3390/geriatrics3030041.

2 Working within a Team

*Pamela L. Steadman-Wood, Kimberly E. Hiroto,
and Harriette Grooh*

"It takes a village"
African proverb

Home Care Teams

Older adults receiving home care generally have complex needs requiring extensive resources. These resources tend to include formal care providers (professionals, paraprofessionals) and informal caregivers (family, friends, and volunteers). Care providers and caregivers vary in their degree of collaboration as a team. High-performing teams are an essential tool in providing effective, patient-centered health care (Mitchell et al., 2012). Team-based health care is defined as "the provision of health services to individuals, families, and/or their communities by at least two health providers who work collaboratively with patients—to accomplish shared goals within and across settings to achieve coordinated, high-quality care" (Mitchell et al., 2012, p. 5). Caring for older adults with complex needs requires an interdisciplinary team (Geriatrics Interdisciplinary Advisory Group, 2006). Health care teams vary in their attitudes, function, and behaviors depending on their degree of integration (Zeiss & Gallagher Thompson, 2003; Zeiss & Steffen, 1996). Multidisciplinary teams tend to have a discipline-specific focus generating independent assessment and treatment plans. Interdisciplinary teams tend to be more integrated, working collaboratively from a comprehensive, biopsychosocial model contributing to assessment and treatment plans.

Factors that impact effective team-based work include the team process, culture, systems, and communication. To work effectively on a home care team, it is important to have a clear understanding of the team's:

- Model of care
- Culture (stakeholders on the team, what services are provided vs. contracted)
- Function (multidisciplinary vs. interdisciplinary)
- Specific roles of each team member

- How to triage, refer, and provide direct care
- Communication regarding patient care and team process (meeting face to face, video conference, teleconference, frequency of meetings; documentation procedures, use of electronic health record, or EHR).

Models of Team-Based Home Care

There are many models of home care teams. In this chapter we draw on examples from the Department of Veterans Affairs (VA) Home-Based Primary Care (HBPC) program, from a private-sector HBPC practice, and from a professional geriatric care management practice: HGA Personal Care Consultants, located in Northern California.

Veterans Affairs Home-Based Primary Care

The Veterans Health Administration developed home care services in 1972 to address the increasing population of Veterans with chronic complex illnesses and associated functional changes (Beales & Edes, 2009). The program aims to maximize Veterans' health, function, and quality of life; minimize the frequency of hospitalizations; and delay nursing home placement (e.g., Beales & Edes, 2009; Karlin & Karel, 2014). Although not specifically focused on older adults, the average age of the HBPC population is 76.5 years (Edes & Burris, 2014). The HBPC program differs from Medicare Home Care services in its scope, breadth, duration of services, and catchment areas (e.g., Beales & Edes, 2009; Edes & Burris, 2014). Efficacy studies demonstrate that HBPC services are associated with reduced admissions to hospitals and nursing homes, decreased lengths of stay, and overall reduced medical costs. The interdisciplinary HBPC team generally includes a physician, nurse practitioner or physician assistant, registered nurses (serving as case managers), pharmacists, dieticians, rehabilitation therapists (e.g., occupational and/or physical therapists), and social workers. In 2007, the VA required that each HBPC team have a full-time doctoral-level mental health (MH) provider on their team, most commonly a psychologist but in some cases a psychiatrist, filling this role. The rationale for specifying a doctoral-level provider focused on the level and type of services often required by Veterans in HBPC (psychotherapy, cognitive, psychodiagnostic assessments, and decisional-capacity assessments; Hicken & Plowhead, 2010; Karlin & Karel, 2014).

Mount Sinai Visiting Doctors Program

The Mount Sinai Visiting Doctors Program (MSVD) is a large interdisciplinary HBPC program that provides care to older adults with complex medical and MH needs (Ornstein, Hernandez, DeCherrie, & Soriano, 2011).

Funded by Mount Sinai Medical Center and private support, MSVD started in 1995 and has become one of the largest academic HBPC programs in the United States (Reckrey et al., 2014), and serves as a major teaching site. The interdisciplinary team consists of physicians, social work case managers, and contracting nursing agencies.

Aging Life Care Professional or Geriatric Care Management

Geriatric care management is another model of home care. The Aging Life Care Association (ALCA), formerly the National Association of Professional Geriatric Care Managers, defines a geriatric care manager (GCM) as "a health and human services specialist who acts as a guide and advocate for families who are caring for older relatives or disabled adults" (ALCA, www.aginglifecare.org/). GCMs assess the client's needs, create a care plan, and coordinate and oversee the care provided. GCMs address needs related to housing, financial management, legal issues, federal and state entitlement benefits, safety, and coordination of medical and MH treatment. These services tend to be private pay, concierge-style services.[1]

One example of a private-sector geriatric consultation and care management (GCCM) team, derived from the Community Mental Health Services Mobile Geriatric Evaluation Team model and adapted from the VA HBPC model, provides integrated home-based services to community-dwelling older adults.[2] The team consists of a geropsychologist and certified care manager, a licensed clinical social worker, an occupational therapist, and registered nurses. Additional advisors include a geriatric psycho-pharmacologist, a geriatric nurse practitioner, and a public benefits/disabilities specialist. The team is experienced in home care, palliative care, and treatment coordination for mental illness and/or substance use. Each team member is specialized in geriatrics and remains dedicated to addressing the complexities of aging.

The MH provider assumes the roles of owner, manager, and supervisor as indicated in Table 2.1.

Table 2.1 Roles of the MH Provider on a GCCM Team

Role	Duties
Owner	• Marketing/promoting the practice • Financial/legal accountability
Manager	• Human resources: recruiting, hiring, firing personnel
Supervisor	• Leadership/oversight • Directing/supporting team members to perform within certain parameters • Intakes; assignment of cases

Cases are assigned a primary and secondary provider based on factors that serve clients' best interests (e.g., skill sets needed, location, and availability). Regardless of pragmatics, team members with skill sets most befitting client needs are assigned as primary or secondary provider. These practical priorities create a GCCM team that provides comprehensive care, as described below.

Mr. Abbott, a 68-year-old single, White, upper-middle-class man with a history of schizophrenia, lives with his sister in their deceased parents' home. After his parents and psychiatrist died six years ago, Mr. Abbott resisted seeking medical and psychiatric help. Police found him disheveled and confused on a roadside and involuntarily hospitalized him. The court appointed a temporary public guardian to oversee involuntary psychiatric treatment. Mr. Abbott's trust officer hired the GCCM team to provide services to the trust officer, Mr. Abbott, and his family. Services included recommending resources for safety and welfare, education and support on the legal process of guardianship and the MH system, advocacy to track his progress through the system, and coordination efforts toward recovery preferably at home. The public guardian provided oversight of the legal process. The MH provider, as the primary care manager, developed a working relationship with Mr. Abbott, and met with the sister, trust officer, and guardian to establish a care plan. The team urged the psychiatric facility to assess his physical and mental health. The team nurse visited regularly, establishing trust with Mr. Abbott to escort him to outpatient appointments. Family visited daily, taking him home for supervised weekend visits. The MH provider attended all case conferences and maintained responsibility for the discharge plan. The MH provider and nurse identified a residential treatment program where he received comprehensive geriatric psychiatric treatment and family counseling. With a greater infrastructure of care, the conservatorship was terminated. The team nurse continued to act as liaison between Mr. Abbott, the facility staff case manager, and the staff nurses during the transition to outpatient care. In preparation for discharge home, the team occupational therapist met with Mr. Abbott, conducted a home safety evaluation, and made recommendations to increase muscle strength and decrease fall risk. The MH provider facilitated outpatient treatment with a psychiatrist and a family therapist. Upon discharge home, the nurse care manager updated the family and trust officer on Mr. Abbott's progress, including assisting with health insurance claims; the social worker helped him apply for public entitlements (e.g., Medicare, Social Security benefits). Eventually, Mr. Abbott's symptoms stabilized, allowing his sister to attend to her own health. With the team's involvement, he maintained therapeutic gains and continued living his life at home as he wished.

Role of the Team-Based MH Provider

The MH provider can serve various roles on a home care team including, but not limited to, direct service provider, consultant, patient advocate, mediator, and educator. Some teams may have MH providers from different disciplines (e.g., social workers, psychologists, psychiatry providers) with occasional role overlap. It is important to negotiate roles and ensure that providers are functioning at the top of their licenses. For example, on teams that have both social workers and psychologists as direct service providers, delineation of roles may be outlined as indicated in Table 2.2.

Consultant

MH providers can serve as consultants and not necessarily provide direct clinical care. The consultant role can vary on home care teams. In some models, the MH provider may conduct a needs assessment for the patient and/or caregiver and coordinate referrals with contracting agencies that

Table 2.2 Example Delineation of Social Worker and Psychologist Roles on a Home Care Team

	Social Worker	*Psychologist*
Assessment	• Initial biopsychosocial assessment • MH screenings (anxiety, depression, cognitive, caregiver burden, etc.) • Community, federal, state, institutional resources	• Psychodiagnostic, psychological, cognitive, decision-making capacity evaluations
Intervention	• Case management • Patient advocacy • Advance directive discussions • Family meetings	• Evidence-based psychotherapy, behavioral health, and caregiver interventions

provide direct services. In other models, the MH provider works collaboratively with team members to provide direct care. For example, a patient may decline MH services but trust the nurse, prompting the nurse to consult the MH provider about patient needs.

Mr. Velazquez is an 85-year-old Latino man living in an in-law apartment upstairs from his daughter and son-in-law. Mr. Velazquez has a neurological condition that affects his balance and mobility, and therefore he has difficulty leaving his home safely. Mr. Velazquez's wife has advanced Alzheimer's disease and resides in a skilled nursing facility. Mr. Velazquez's daughter and son-in-law work full-time and are away from home most of the day. They hired a home care team to help Mr. Velazquez continue living independently. The home care team includes Mr. Velazquez's daughter, a nurse, an MH provider, and a home health aide (HHA). The nurse visiting Mr. Velazquez every two weeks noticed changes over the past couple of months: he became more isolated, with reduced appetite and decreased interest in activities he once enjoyed (reading the paper, chatting about current events). The nurse asked Mr. Velazquez if he would consider talking to the MH provider, but he declined, stating, "You don't need to worry about me, this is what happens when you get old." The nurse consulted the MH provider, who made the following recommendations: administer the Geriatric Depression Scale-short (15-item) and the California Older Person's Pleasant Events Schedule (COPPES), and obtain collateral information from Mr. Velazquez's daughter (with his permission). Mr. Velazquez's responses on the GDS-s suggested clinical depression. He endorsed interest in 30/66 activities on the COPPES but did not think he would be able to engage in them. Due to her increasing work demands, Mr. Velazquez's daughter had meals delivered to him, rather than eating breakfast with him, and no longer drove him to visit his wife. The nurse and MH provider devised a treatment plan to include: (1) hanging a bird feeder outside Mr. Velazquez's window with a local bird identification chart, (2) having the HHA serve his breakfast and read the newspaper with him three days per week, and (3) arranging for Mr. Velazquez to have dinner with his wife three nights per week. After one month, Mr. Velazquez no longer endorsed depressive symptoms, and his daughter and caregivers reported that he was "back to his old self."

Facilitator

MH providers have specialized training in effective communication, conflict resolution, and group and individual therapy. As such, the provider may be in the role of facilitating team processing. For example, they may help the team process grief, cope with conflict, resolve challenging patient care situations, and manage job-related stressors. While this can be a rewarding role for the provider, it can be challenging to serve in dual roles as team member and team facilitator.

> A nurse approached Dr. Patel, the team psychologist, about the nurse's grief since a patient died. The team did not have a formal process for addressing loss. Dr. Patel met with the nurse several times and provided empathic listening. Over time, he grew uncomfortable as the content of their meetings bordered on individual therapy. Dr. Patel spoke to the program manager and suggested a monthly team support meeting for processing emotions related to the challenges of their work. The group was well received by staff.

Triaging Referrals

In addition to delineating roles, it is important to develop a referral process for MH issues. Some questions to consider in the referral process include:

- How are patients' MH needs identified and addressed?
- Is there a formal screening process? Are MH issues raised during treatment planning meetings, on regularly scheduled visits, etc.?
- Does the MH provider need to see every referral?
- What is the triage process?
- How are assessments and treatment outcomes communicated to the team?

On integrated teams, the MH provider may attend all treatment planning meetings and contribute directly to the treatment plan. On less integrated teams, all disciplines may document in the patient's record independently. Establishing a system to communicate among team members is vital to ensure all care needs are met.

Addressing Performance Measures

Depending on the organization, certain MH-related performance measures may be monitored. Examples include screenings for depression, suicidal ideation, and substance use. Often these clinical screenings are a shared responsibility; it behooves the team to identify who owns these tasks.

Education

Depending on the teams' familiarity of MH services, MH providers may need to provide education on their role and services provided. Ongoing team training and education helps team members learn about the services of each discipline.

Facilitating Team Functioning

As described above, the role of the MH provider on home care teams is often multifold (e.g., direct care provider, consultant, facilitator) and extends to addressing the needs of the team as well. This may involve providing team training on relevant issues (e.g., interpersonal boundaries, mental illness, cultural sensitivity). Although providers on home care teams often work with older adults and/or those with disabilities, the providers themselves may not have specialty training to work with these populations. The MH provider may observe gaps in the team's knowledge base or training that he/she may help fill. They may also offer to work with the program manager to develop educational in-services on relevant topics within their area of expertise. Additionally, team members may not be familiar working with MH providers or other disciplines on the team. Joint visits with other team members allow them to see each other in action, understand how services complement each other, and promote collaborative teamwork.

Issues Facing Home Care Teams

Professional Boundaries

Home care services often provide long-term care to their patients, allowing providers to follow patients through their life course, including death. One of the most common challenges for such teams involves professional and interpersonal boundaries (Hicken & Plowhead, 2010; Sanders, Bullock, & Broussard, 2012). The intimacy of providing home care can foster a sense of over-familiarity, which can lead to boundary violations and ethical drift. Providing home care to under-resourced or seriously ill individuals can foster a sense of fulfillment within the team, but it can also tempt team members to go above and beyond. While often well-intentioned, these extra efforts can set a precedent that the team finds unsustainable and can lead to compassion fatigue and/or burnout if staff feel, for example, that patient needs continually exceed their professional bandwidth. Addressing these and other common challenges in home care often contributes to improved team functioning and sustainability.

Dr. Clarke, the psychologist on the home-based care team, received word from a colleague that one of the nurses had been purchasing groceries for Mr. Smith, an 85-year-old African American homebound patient without access to transportation. He reportedly entrusted this nurse with his debit card. Concerned about ethics and interpersonal and professional boundaries, Dr. Clarke inquired further with this nurse, who openly acknowledged helping Mr. Smith and viewed this as "going the extra mile." This nurse also described praying with Mr. Smith and helping with light housework during her visit, which she reported other nurses also did. Dr. Clarke explored the underlying meaning and value for this nurse of "going the extra mile," which related to her cultural and professional caregiver identity and her affection for older adults. However, the nurse's narrative also revealed a negative view of aging focused on loss, and her actions seemed somewhat motivated by pity. With the program manager's permission, Dr. Clarke and the social worker conducted in-services on professional boundaries including ethics, behavioral dos and don'ts, and education on the risks to team integrity and patient trust when boundaries are violated. Dr. Clarke acknowledged that personal and regional cultures influence staff interactions with older adults at home and addressed these norms while focusing on patient preferences (e.g., how patients wish to be addressed). Dr. Clarke also partnered with the rehabilitation therapists to present the aging process from a strength-based perspective with themes of resiliency, personhood, and autonomy. As for Mr. Smith, he accepted a food delivery service allowing him to select his groceries, and a vanpool that transports him to church. These interventions increased his autonomy, re-established interpersonal boundaries, and increased his socialization with his faith community.

MH providers are trained to attend to interpersonal and professional boundaries, although helping interdisciplinary teams do the same can be challenging. Disciplines may vary in their definition of professional boundaries, but most assert that the provider must respect their position of power relative to the patient, prevent dual relationships, and ensure that their interpersonal relationship does not harm the patient (e.g., American Psychological Association, 2017; National Association of Social Workers, 2010). Boundary violations may be insidious or occur abruptly: a nurse may develop romantic feelings toward the adult child of a patient, resulting in frequent visits to the patient's home; another provider may drive a patient to the store as a good deed. With the increasing instrumental needs of an aging population with comorbid conditions, it is not uncommon for the MH provider or team members to be pulled to engage in housework, grocery shopping, and pet management outside their scope of practice. Some team members may want two different patients to become roommates, to provide peer support and mutual caregiving, and want to introduce them to one another. Other team members may want to introduce their family members to the patient, feeling a close rapport as home care evolves. Some team members may want to disregard indications that are contrary to safe and effective provision of home care, such as threatening behavior, reasoning that the patient's best chance at medical care is via home care. Finally, team members may insist that another team member implement a specific treatment, such as psychotherapy or physical therapy, not accepting that the patient and family have refused to consent to these specific services. The earlier these boundary violations are noticed and addressed, the easier they are to remedy.

Finding teachable moments within the team can help create a culture that values and consistently practices professional boundaries. The MH provider may present on professional boundaries as part of the orientation to new hires, model self-reflective practice around boundaries, and find moments within team discussions to highlight the importance of boundaries. Having specific policies regarding these issues, and reviewing the Health Insurance Portability and Accountability Act or other laws within this context, can be helpful to ensure appropriate care.

Burnout and Compassion Fatigue

Maintaining appropriate boundaries also helps prevent burnout and compassion fatigue. Burnout is often associated with systemic challenges (e.g., managing bureaucracy, inadequate leadership) and a limited sense of personal/professional value or accomplishment. Compassion fatigue, however, is often associated with vicarious trauma and the effect of prolonged empathic engagement with trauma survivors (Figley, 2002; McCann & Pearlman, 1990). It may manifest as anxiety, social withdrawal, depression, and a reduced sense of safety, trust, or power. Compassion fatigue can apply to nurses and other team members in addition to MH providers and first responders, as originally intended. Patients often confide in non-MH team members, making them the holders of this information without formal ways of processing it. Attention to both burnout and compassion fatigue within the team is important given the population served in home care and the systemic challenges of doing this work.

Bearing witness to situations often encountered in home visits (e.g., abject poverty, suspected abuse, failure to thrive) can elicit sincere empathy, a sense of helplessness, and frustration with systems that struggle to support patient needs. Given their training, MH providers are well suited to address the risks for burnout and compassion fatigue. Acknowledging the problem can validate team members' struggles and humanity. Highlighting ways the team positively impacted the patient and family can help increase the team's self-efficacy, and explaining how to manage difficult personalities may improve team members' communication strategies. Similarly, encouraging and modeling self-care and help-seeking may support team members struggling with compassion fatigue. Other strategies may include protecting time to discuss the team's frustrations and struggles, celebrating moments of success, and offering support during times of emotional pain.

Grief and Bereavement

Providing long-term care to homebound patients often includes bearing witness to their end-of-life. Like any person, home care providers may grieve when patients die. Creating emotional space to process grief is important to honor the relationship, process the loss, and support team members' return to work. While not serving as an individual therapist, the MH provider can provide empathic listening and, if necessary, recommend further support services. The MH provider themselves may openly process their emotions, giving others permission to do the same. Teams may also develop ways of honoring the deceased (e.g., sending bereavement cards to family, developing rituals to memorialize patients). Helping the team heal each other's wounds and process difficult discussions can foster trust, build resiliency, and increase sustainability.

Implicit Bias

Working with primarily older adults involves confronting our own biases of aging, disability, illness, class, and other aspects of diversity and intersectionality. *Implicit bias* refers to one's individual and collective sociocultural history that can affect attitudes and behaviors at a level below self-awareness (e.g., Greenwald & Banaji, 1995). Ageism is one of the few "-isms" that remains socially acceptable in society (e.g., birthday cards, anti-aging advertisements). As products of our culture and society, we all have implicit biases and must acknowledge our responsibility to address them. When they go unacknowledged, implicit biases can manifest as microaggressions: subtle statements or behaviors that (unintentionally) imply ignorance, negative views, and/or hostility toward a particular group (Sue et al., 2007). Although initially applied to racism, microaggressions also apply to ageism and the intersection of age with other cultural factors.

Although many geriatrics providers are mindful of ageism, implicit biases and microaggressions still surface. Individuals must be aware of and address these biases within themselves and others without judgment or guilt, lest they become a toxic blind spot. Negative ageist biases in health care providers can affect patient care through delayed treatment (Levy & Meyers, 2004), lowered expectations for improvement (Lamberty & Bares, 2013), and assumptions that older adults cannot change (Kane, 2004). Internalized ageism within patients can affect their performance on cognitive tests (Levy, Zonderman, Slade, & Ferrucci, 2012), physical function, and decisions around life-sustaining treatments (Levy, Slade, & Kasl, 2002). Recall the example of Dr. Clarke earlier in this chapter. The psychologist noticed the nurse's tendency to view aging in a negative light. Rather than holding the nurse accountable, the psychologist provided in-services and emphasized a strength-based approach to aging. Offering formal training on aging and its intersection with other cultural variables, including mental illness, can help correct and broaden team members' perspectives and invite further discussion. Informal approaches to addressing ageist microaggressions can also help shape team culture and gently challenge biases without shaming team members. For example, a team member may describe a patient as "adorable" and "cute." The MH provider, aware of the patient's struggles to assert their autonomy and personhood, may note how these terms inadvertently belittle the patient and diminish their individuality. The provider may try to broaden the team member's view of the patient by describing the patient's life experiences and resiliency, and perhaps even disclosing (if clinically appropriate) the patient's struggle to be seen as more than an older adult. This approach ideally will not shame or call-out the team member, but instead focus on the patient's experience and refocus the team's goal of providing patient-centered care.

Helping to develop a team culture that engages in difficult conversations, reflects on their process, and tolerates distress creates a foundation for discussing issues like implicit biases and cultural diversity. The MH provider can model how to discuss implicit biases by reflecting on their own (as appropriate and psychologically safe) and can depersonalize the process by framing common collective biases as artifacts of our society. However, such discussions are delicate and depend on team members' own cultural identity development, diversity awareness, and recognition of their power and privilege relative to others. Additionally, the initiator and messenger of this information may count. Depending on the MH provider's stimulus value to the team, they may or may not be the most appropriate person to facilitate a discussion on these topics.

Summary

Providing integrated home care services to older adults can be both rewarding and challenging. MH providers take on many roles within the team and are often trained with the skills to enhance team functioning. A cohesive, knowledgeable, and trusting team is the key to doing this work successfully and achieving the best outcomes for the patient, families, and home care staff. While achieving this often takes time, the MH provider can make significant contributions to affect team functioning and improve the lives of home care patients.

Notes

1 For more in-depth discussion of other models of care management teams, please see www.aginglifecarejournal.org/providing-care-management-with-a-multidisciplinary-team-managing-quality/.
2 See www.hgapersonalcareconsultants.com.

References

American Psychological Association. (2017). *Ethical principles of psychologists and code of conduct*. Washington, DC: Author.
Beales, J. L., & Edes, T. (2009). Veteran's affairs home based primary care. *Clinical Geriatric Medicine, 25*, 149–154. doi:10.1016/j.cger.2008.11.002.
Edes, T., & Burris, J. F. (2014). Home-based primary care: A VA innovation coming soon. *Physician Leadership Journal, 1*, 38–42.
Figley, C. R. (2002). Compassion fatigue: Psychotherapists' chronic lack of self care. *Journal of Clinical Psychology/In Session: Psychotherapy in Practice, 58*, 1433–1441. doi:10.1002/jclp.10090.
Geriatrics Interdisciplinary Advisory Group. (2006). Interdisciplinary care for older adults with complex needs: American Geriatrics Society position statement. *Journal of the American Geriatrics Society, 54*, 849–852. doi:10.1111/j.1532.2006.00707.x.
Greenwald, A. G., & Banaji, M. R. (1995). Implicit social cognition: Attitudes, self-esteem, and stereotypes. *Psychological Review, 102*, 4–27.
Hicken, B. L., & Plowhead, A. (2010). A model for home-based psychology from the Veterans Health Administration. *Professional Psychology: Research and Practice, 41*, 340–346. doi:10.1037/a0020431.
Kane, M. N. (2004). Ageism and intervention: What social work students believe about training people differently because of age. *Educational Gerontology, 30*, 767–784. doi:10.1080/0360127490498098.
Karlin, B., & Karel, M. J. (2014). National integration of mental health providers in VA home-based primary care: A innovative model for mental health care delivery with older. *The Gerontologist, 54*, 1–12. doi:10.1093/geront/gnt142.
Lamberty, G. L., & Bares, K. K. (2013). Neuropsychological assessment and management of older adults with multiple somatic symptoms. In L. D. Ravdin & H. L. Katzen (Eds.), *Handbook on the neuropsychology of aging and dementia* (pp. 121–134). New York, NY: Springer.

Levy, B. R., & Meyers, L. M. (2004). Preventive health behaviors influenced by self-perceptions of aging. *Preventive Medicine, 39*, 625–629. doi:10.1016/j. ypmed.2004.02.029.

Levy, B. R., Slade, S., & Kasl, S. (2002). Longitudinal benefit of positive self-perceptions of aging on functional health. *Journal of Gerontology: Psychological Science, 57*, 409–417. doi:10.1093/geronb/57.5.P409.

Levy, B. R., Zonderman, A. B., Slade, M. D., & Ferrucci, L. (2012). Memory shaped by age stereotypes over time. *Journal of Gerontology: Psychological Science, 67*, 432–436. doi:10.1093/geronb/gbr120.

McCann, I. L., & Pearlman, L. A. (1990). Vicarious traumatization: A framework for understanding the psychological effects of working with victims. *Journal of Traumatic Stress, 3*, 131–149.

Mitchell, P., Wynia, M., Golden, R., McNellis, B., Okun, S., Webb, C. E., & Von Kohorn, I. (2012). *Core principles & values of effective team-based health care.* Presented at the Washington, DC. Retrieved fromhttps://nam.edu/wp-content/uploads/2015/06/VSRT-Team-Based-Care-Principles-Values.pdf.

National Association of Social Workers. (2010). *Code of ethics.* Washington, DC: Author.

Ornstein, K., Hernandez, C. R., DeCherrie, L. V., & Soriano, T. A. (2011). The Mount Sinai (NewYork) Visiting Doctors Program: Meeting the needs of the urban homebound population. *Care Management Journals: Journal of Case Management, 12*, 159–163.

Reckrey, J. M., Gettenberg, G. G., Ross, H., Kopke, V., Soriano, T., & Ornstein, K. (2014). The critical role of social workers in home-based primary care. *Social Work Health Care, 53*, 330–343. doi:10.1080/00981389.2014.884041.

Sanders, S., Bullock, K., & Broussard, C. (2012). Exploring professional boundaries in end-of-life care: Considerations for hospice social workers and other members of the team. *Journal of Social Work in End-of-Life & Palliative Care, 8*, 10–28. doi:10.108-/15524256.2012.650671.

Sue, D. W., Capodilupo, C. M., Torino, G. C., Bucceri, J. M., Holder, A. M., Nadal, K. L., & Esquilin, M. (2007). Racial microaggressions in everyday life. Implications for clinical practice. *American Psychologist, 62*, 271–286. doi:10.1037/0003-066X.62.4.271.

Zeiss, A. M., & Gallagher Thompson, D. (2003). Providing interdisciplinary geriatric team care: What does it really take? *Clinical Psychology: Science and Practice, 10*, 115–119. doi:10.1093/clinpsy.10.1.115.

Zeiss, A. M., & Steffen, A. (1996). Interdisciplinary health care teams: The basic unit of geriatric care. In Carstensen, L. L., Edelstein, B. A., & Dornbrand, L. (Eds.). *The practical handbook of clinical gerontology* (pp. 423–450). Thousand Oaks, CA: Sage Publications.

3 Establishing and Maintaining a Therapeutic Relationship

Janet Yang, Marc Parker, and Carlos Santell

Conducting assessment and psychotherapy with patients in their homes presents numerous clinical, ethical, legal, and practical issues. This chapter highlights suggestions for mental health (MH) providers establishing a psychotherapeutic relationship with persons in their homes. Specifically, this chapter will address establishing rapport, setting the therapeutic frame, establishing treatment direction, addressing cultural differences, managing shifts in ongoing rapport, and dealing with transference. The authors draw on experience working at Heritage Clinic, a community-based MH agency in a large urban city, which serves older adults, most of whom are of low income and diverse cultural backgrounds.

Mrs. Johns was a 73-year-old Caucasian woman who was referred to Heritage Clinic by her primary care provider due to symptoms of complicated grief and trauma. Mrs. Johns reported the death of her mother two years earlier to Alzheimer's disease, the death of a neighbor in a shooting, and ongoing conflict with her adult daughter, with whom she lived. Mrs. Johns attended psychotherapy 10 years ago, for about a year, which facilitated relief from guilt she felt for placing her mother in a facility. Mrs. Johns often missed health care appointments due to fatigue and social anxiety, and stated she preferred in-home sessions.

Early sessions focused on developing rapport, and her MH provider commented on Mrs. Johns' cats as they entered the living room. The provider accepted a bottle of water that she offered. Mrs. Johns identified that her goal was to "get back to where I was two years ago." She wanted to increase the frequency of attending medical appointments, go out with friends more frequently, and let go of resentment that she felt towards her daughter. Mrs. Johns refused psychiatric medication, due to fear of complications with medications that she took for a seizure disorder. Mrs. Johns also expressed shame about meeting her provider in her pajamas, and about her frequent tearfulness. The provider provided empathy and validation about Mrs. Johns' conflicts with her daughter and encouraged her to identify what she found most helpful about her previous psychotherapy.

Six weeks into therapy, Mrs. Johns abruptly canceled a session because her daughter was home from work, and Mrs. Johns didn't want her to know she was in psychotherapy. In the weeks after, her daughter began working from home more frequently, which made scheduling sessions at home difficult. The MH provider offered Mrs. Johns three possible solutions: they could have telephone sessions on those days that her daughter was present, meet at a local library, or, knowing that one of Mrs. Johns' goals was to attend more medical appointments, they could begin to meet in the clinic. With some hesitation, Mrs. Johns agreed to the latter.

About three months later, Mrs. Johns continued to attend weekly sessions in the clinic. She reported pride that she had been changing out of her pajamas and getting out of the house more frequently. Mrs. Johns identified that had her initial sessions not been in the home, had she not gotten to meet the MH provider and felt heard, she doubted that she would have felt up to coming to the clinic.

Establishing Rapport

As illustrated in the above vignette, an MH treatment relationship begins with establishing rapport. Rapport-building starts before the first visit and can be facilitated in a variety of ways. With older adults, rapport can be enhanced by gaining knowledge and awareness of age-related concepts, such as developmental aging effects, cohort influences, retirement, widowhood, illness, and disability issues. Rapport can also be facilitated in advance by gathering information from the referral source and the patient, and by beginning to form hypotheses about the best approach for the patient. Did the patient refer himself or herself, and is the patient likely to jump right in for psychotherapy? Or, if a third party has referred this patient, is he or she assenting to services? If so, the patient may be ambivalent. As in the vignette about Mrs. Johns, who had had psychotherapy before, the initial approach could be more straightforward in starting psychotherapy with a thorough MH assessment and formation of a psychotherapeutic treatment plan.

Handling Ambivalence

When a new patient is ambivalent about psychotherapy, it may be necessary to start therapy more slowly and be more flexible throughout the therapy process. For example, when a patient has been referred by his daughter, but he does not think he needs psychotherapy ("I'm not crazy!"), it may be helpful to start by talking with the patient about a topic of mutual interest (e.g., a local sports team) or about how he feels about his daughter thinking he needs MH services, rather than quickly moving to a formal psychological assessment. Ambivalence, or even disinterest in therapy, is common following referrals from outside agencies like Adult Protective Services (APS). For example, when a referral is received from APS that a woman is malnourished, the provider can talk with the APS social worker to determine what the patient thinks is a problem, if any. The potential patient may think the problem is that APS is bothering her. Thus, an initial approach might be to empathize with the patient about the troublesome social worker.

Collaboration

Collaborating with or referencing community partners can enhance early rapport. It can be helpful to verbally reference community partners during interactions, or to make a team visit to the patient, when the other partners have pre-established relationships. In Mrs. Johns' case, noting that her doctor had suggested therapy enhanced trust. The provider can ask the referral source what type of relationship he or she has with the patient. If the relationship seems positive, the provider can mention the referring person (such as "Alice Moore, the social worker from your hospital, let me know that you had told her you were missing your husband. Can you tell me more about that?"). If the relationship seems to be strained or negative, it may be best to avoid mentioning it. For example, if the referring party is an apartment complex manager who has noticed that the patient is angry and starts arguments in the complex, it may be wiser to avoid mentioning what the manager told you.

Listening

Careful listening, empathy, compassion, and validation of the patient's point of view are critical. Listening may begin by empathizing with overt feelings and meaning. For example, when the patient says she misses her husband, you could say, "That must be sad." However, listening can also involve attending to deeper meanings. A patient with dementia may say, "I want to go to work," and an empathic response might be "It sounds like you really would like to be more useful these days." Patients with altered views of reality can be particularly challenging to empathize with and validate. For patients with a psychotic disorder, it may be best to empathize with the feelings while not challenging the misperceptions (Yang, Garis, Jackson, & McClure, 2009). For example, when a patient with delusions says, "The neighbors are infiltrating my air conditioning," it may be helpful to say, "It sounds like that must be frightening" (or "... make you angry," depending on what emotions he or she is indicating), and withhold the impulse to say, "How could they be doing that?"

Using Appropriate Titles

At the start of the treatment relationship, consider using titles to address the patient (Mr., Mrs., Ms., Dr., Rev., etc.). This can show respect and enhance rapport, as well as enhancing trust and self-esteem. For example, if the patient is a retired college professor who gained self-esteem through her professional position, calling her by her first name could feel belittling, while calling her "Dr. Smith" could suggest to her that the provider values her life experience. Switch to using the patient's first name if the patient suggests doing so, or the provider may ask the patient what he or she wants to be called. With older patients, it is often appropriate to continue using the title throughout therapy.

It can also be helpful for the provider to consider whether or not to use their title ahead of his or her name, depending on whether he or she wants to emphasize formality or informality. For example, if the patient seems to be hesitant to engage in professional services, leaving out the title might facilitate rapport. Or, if the provider perceives the patient may have difficulties with boundaries (e.g., a patient with a Borderline Personality Disorder) using his or her title might help emphasize the professionalism of the encounters.

Using the Environment

A benefit of home care is that the provider can use the physical environment to understand some of what is meaningful to the patient, and use these observations to help build rapport. In addition, the act of going into another person's home can also aid in rapport-building, as it necessitates a closeness and comfort, unlike outpatient settings. Consider Mrs. Johns, who indicated that she would not have come to the clinic at the start of therapy. The MH provider may notice personal affects or items in the home that may be meaningful to the patient. They may also notice artwork, greeting cards, or trinkets, and engage the patient in a discussion about those items. As with Mrs. Johns, the provider can comment on, interact with, or (if not allergic) stroke a pet and show pleasure in it.

With more reticent patients, continuing to talk about external objects may be easier to discuss than psychological symptoms and issues. However, the MH provider should watch for signs that commenting on personal belongings might feel intrusive to the patient. For example, the provider might notice photographs of young children on the wall and comment on what he or she thinks are the patient's grandchildren. If the patient reacts with silence or withdrawal, it may be that the patient does not want to think or talk about this subject. Therefore, carefully selecting the pieces of information that one comments on or interacts with can maximize the impact on rapport-building.

When coming into a patient's home, a wealth of information is available regarding their personal issues and practical needs. In Mrs. Johns' case, the MH provider became aware that she tended to stay in her pajamas, which would likely not be evident in the clinic. As a provider becomes aware of practical needs, he or she needs to decide what response is likely to be most clinically helpful. It may be that helping a patient with a practical need is a useful method of developing rapport. For example, if the patient is clearly unable to cook, establishing dietary assistance (like Meals on Wheels) could both improve the patient's well-being and enhance rapport. Or, if the provider notices the patient's home is in significant disrepair, referral to a low-cost home repair agency could help develop the therapeutic relationship. A wise MH provider will assess for, and consider helping with, practical needs, while not moving too quickly, which may undermine independence. Helping the patient and the developing rapport should be considered in the context of enhancing patients' personal empowerment rather than enabling dependency. This will be discussed further below.

Setting the Therapeutic Frame

One of the significant challenges of conducting psychotherapy in a patient's home is setting a professional, therapeutic framework (Yang et al., 2009). The home is more informal and less controlled than an office or clinic setting. Unlike outpatient work, there are many more decisions to be made in setting the context and frame. The MH provider needs to consider how to act professionally and establish the boundaries of a patient–therapist relationship, while at the same time being flexible enough with the circumstances to invite the development of an empathic relationship.

Clothing

It is important for the provider to be seen as a professional, but also as someone who is approachable and relatable. Weighing how formally versus informally to present oneself may vary based on several patient considerations. For example, when going to visit a patient who is known to engage in hoarding behaviors, the provider may dress more casually, in washable clothes. Contrast this with a patient who is a recently retired professional; the provider's dress may mirror the patient's previous working environment. Most often, it is appropriate to dress in business-casual attire, as excessively formal attire may present a stiff and detached impression. In addition, clothing will often need to be practical, given the additional elements that one may contend with on a typical day (see Chapter 6).

Time Frame

One way in which psychotherapy is distinguished from friendly visiting is timing. Traditional, in-office therapy sessions are usually 45 minutes to an hour and start and end promptly; many therapy offices' clocks are easily visible to the MH provider. To mimic these elements, adhering to a set time will help orient the therapeutic interaction towards a professional interaction. It might also be helpful for the provider to state how long the sessions are expected to last (e.g., "I expect our visits to each last about 50 minutes."). The provider should come prepared with a watch or other timepiece that can be easily viewed. However, unanticipated occurrences may require some flexibility with time. For example, when starting a session, if the patient has to use the bathroom and is slow to ambulate, the provider may decide to extend the session.

Confidentiality and Managing Others

It is important to consider how to respond to interruptions during the encounter. An MH provider will want to prepare for the presence of family members, or for the patient receiving a visitor (e.g., home health aide, neighbor, letter carrier) during the session. This may include discussing how you will handle these interruptions, or even discontinuing a session if there are significant concerns related to confidentiality.

Setting the frame includes establishing privacy to talk with the intended patient, and potentially involving family members or other caregivers when appropriate. As indicated with Mrs. Johns, when her daughter was in the home it became more difficult to conduct sessions. While there are numerous factors to consider, one approach to determine whether to include others may to be to observe the patient and family members during the first session, using this as an assessment of the overall context. Later, the provider can assertively state the need for privacy for future sessions.

It is critical to have some time alone with the patient during the first few sessions to assess for issues, feelings, or concerns the patient may not state in front of significant others. The MH provider should voice to all stakeholders that privacy in therapy is essential. Asking the patient, when he or she is in the presence of family members, whether he or she wants family members to leave can put the patient in an awkward position, which may have later repercussions, such as anger or hurt feelings. If the MH provider states this as a need for the treatment, the patient is less likely to feel pressured, and the family is less likely to direct hurt or anger at the patient. Establishing privacy can be done by sitting in a more private room, or by asking other persons present to leave. As indicated in Mrs. Johns' case, when the relationship had progressed further, privacy could be established by inviting the patient to come to the clinic.

Expectations Related to Food and Drink

It is also important to consider ahead of time how to respond to offers of food or drink. Accepting offers of food or drink may enhance rapport-building, as with Mrs. Johns, but it also may dilute the professionalism of the interaction. It may be best to initially respond with a gentle refusal of food or drink offers to set a more professional tone, but allow flexibility to enhance rapport. An MH provider will also want to consider cultural factors, where refusal of the patient's hospitality may be understood as offensive and it is more beneficial to accept. Cultural differences will be discussed further below.

Setting up Expectations and Informed Consent

Many older adult patients are having their first experience in psychotherapy. Therefore, the MH provider should be prepared to describe what psychotherapy is. This can include explaining what the patient is expected to do or talk about, what the therapist will do, how long each session will last, how long the sessions will continue, what any family members are expected (or not expected) to do, and what payments are necessary. The content of this psychoeducation will vary depending on the provider's therapeutic approach. During this discussion, it will be helpful to elicit the expectations of the patient and any family members who are present, and to take their expectations into consideration, while holding certain essential therapeutic boundaries. In describing the therapeutic process, the provider will need to decide whether to use more professional and formal language, which might be the case for patients who are less ambivalent and of a Western culture, or whether to use more informal language, which might be best for more ambivalent patients, and patients of cultures that are less familiar with psychotherapy.

Establishing Who Is Responsible for Therapy

When setting the frame for psychotherapy, it is important to not "over function" for the patient. Home-based therapy requires that the provider set up the appointment and drive to the patient's home. Before that first meeting, the provider has unintentionally introduced a work imbalance that can be counterproductive for therapy. When providers go to a patient rather than requiring the patient go to them, it can lower the investment and motivation for therapy, may impact their preparation or engagement during sessions, or alter their appointment attendance. In other words, it can be important to find ways to support the patient's engagement in therapy, to set boundaries, or even consider termination when it is clear that patients are only participating because the provider showed up to their house.

The provider may also overstep with patients due to the way in which providers might be treated in the home. It is possible to feel more like a family member or friend, and this can pull for the provider to take care of the patient, when longer-term goals may be to increase independence. Being aware of this potential dynamic, and avoiding "rescuing" patients, can help to avoid these pitfalls. Patients may also ask for assistance with non-therapeutic tasks, like rides to their doctor's appointments or other household chores. Given that most therapeutic approaches aim to increase independence rather than reliance on the provider, giving in to these requests can be counterproductive. Saying no may require the provider to tolerate feelings of anxiety or the patient's anger, in the service of longer-term growth of the patient. A discerning provider will problem-solve for those patients who are unable to meet needs on their own, while promoting self-sufficiency in those patients who are more capable themselves.

Establishing Treatment Direction

Similar to the outpatient clinic setting, when beginning treatment at home the provider will collaborate with the patient to establish treatment goals. In the home, the MH provider is more likely to become aware of practical, psychological, medical, and other needs, and may have to prioritize goals differently. The provider should collaborate with the patient to establish short- and long-term goals. It can be helpful to ask the patient, "What would you like to get out of our time together?" or "What would you like to see different in your life in six months, or one year, from now?" It is also important for the provider to make his or her own assessment of needs that the patient may not verbalize. For example, it may become apparent that the patient is not receiving adequate food or taking care of medical needs, or there may be unmet safety, housing, financial, substance-use, or spiritual needs. In addition to working directly to help the patient towards the patient's stated goals, the provider may also incorporate a Motivational Interviewing (Miller & Rollnick, 1991) approach to help the patient towards health goals that the patient may not yet have the energy or insight to approach. When family members are involved, the provider may listen to the family's wishes, and then discuss the family's perspective with the patient individually to determine if the patient agrees with the family's desires. When there are multiple complex problems, it can help to prioritize them and work on one or two goals at a time, and not try to address more than that at any one time. Thinking of Maslow's Hierarchy of Needs (Maslow, 1943) may be a helpful heuristic to consider when prioritizing goals.

MH providers are mandated reporters, and a provider may witness something that requires reporting to APS or Child Protective Services. Navigating the patient's goals, the family's motivation, and the provider's legal and ethical responsibility in such cases can be difficult, and such cases may call for careful consultation and supervision.

Addressing Cultural Differences

Certain cultural issues may be particularly salient in patients' homes, and a culturally competent MH provider will address cultural differences. Upon receiving the referral, prior to visiting the home the provider should note the patient's sociodemographic characteristics, such as age, ethnicity, race, religion, and LGBT status.

Once in the home, it is important to take time to discuss cultural preferences with the patient, demonstrate an interest in knowing their points of view, and try to see the problems from the patient's cultural perspective. For example, one MH provider worked with an East Asian American older adult patient who, after a small heart attack, decided to move in with her daughter. The patient expressed feeling worried about going to live with her daughter and not with her son. When the provider asked for more details, the patient explained that, according to her culture, the male children, especially the eldest son, are expected to take charge of their aging parents. Showing curiosity in this way facilitates understanding the patient's point of view and his or her motives for actions based on culture. When addressing patient actions in the home from a cultural perspective, the provider might ask a question such as, "What does it mean to you that you decided to do that?" or "What does it mean in your culture that you chose to do that?"

Following the initial greeting, the provider should observe behaviors that may carry cultural meaning. For example, the provider may note who goes first through the door of the home, or who accompanies a patient to the exit door. Multiple pairs of shoes may be observed at the entrance to the home, indicating whether there may be a cultural expectation of removing one's shoes; this can be a natural sign of respect and consideration and thereby facilitate rapport.

Showing sensitivity to how the patient moves or acts, and asking questions about meaning and cultural significance, can help the rapport development, ensuring that cultural beliefs are respected and considered. Observing images or pictures inside the home can help to evaluate the patient's spirituality or religion, or other culturally meaningful issues. MH providers can also listen for spiritual phrases of the older adult and consider whether they can be addressed to strengthen rapport.

In the homes of patients in some collectivistic cultures (e.g., Latino, African American, or Middle Eastern American), there may be more family involvement and greater probability of needing to address the presence of other family members in the session.

Working in the home with an older adult with an LGBT identity may offer particular aids to rapport development. For example, the provider may show interest and ask how close the patient feels to a caregiver, long-term roommate, or partner of the same gender, and thereby facilitate the patient sharing more about her or his sexual orientation.

Managing Shifts in Rapport

Mr. Martin was a 72-year-old African American man who received home-based MH and case management services for 18 months. Mr. Martin had MH diagnoses of major depressive disorder and generalized anxiety disorder, and he was undergoing chemotherapy for cancer throughout this time. Mr. Martin experienced sadness, hopelessness, and anger about having cancer, which contributed to non-adherence to medical treatment and social isolation.

Mr. Martin was seen in his home by his MH provider and by a case manager, who was linking him to supportive services. He frequently ended sessions after 30–35 minutes, stating that he was in too much pain or feeling sick from chemotherapy. Mr. Martin had some success in meeting his goals of increased socialization and consistent attendance of medical appointments, which he attributed to good relationships with his MH provider and case manager.

During one appointment, Mr. Martin's case manager found him in bed and complaining of intense stomach pain. Mr. Martin reported that he had skipped his chemotherapy appointment earlier that day, and he stated that he was too sick to meet. The case manager, assessing that he was in imminent danger, called 911 on Mr. Martin's behalf and convinced him to go with paramedics to the hospital. A couple hours later, Mr. Martin's MH provider called him to check in. Mr. Martin reported that he was sent home after a brief examination. Angrily, he stated, "I told you it wouldn't do any good!"

Mr. Martin called the office to cancel his next psychotherapy session on the day of the appointment, when the provider was already en route to his home. Mr. Martin invited the provider inside and expressed anger that no one had listened to him: the case manager, paramedics, emergency room doctor, and the MH provider. Mr. Martin ended the session after 15 minutes, but he agreed to meet with the provider the next week.

After the 911 call, Mr. Martin's engagement with sessions was inconsistent. He didn't answer calls, turned his MH provider away at his door, and ended sessions earlier than usual, stating that he felt sick. Mr. Martin denied feeling angry since shortly after the 911 call, and he was reluctant to discuss that event further.

While establishing rapport is primarily a task at the beginning of psychotherapy, rapport must continue to be nurtured, and at times re-established after a breach in the therapeutic relationship. Because home-based care may expose reportable (e.g., safety) or medically emergent situations, providers may be required to act against the wishes of the patient. Sometimes patients struggle to re-engage with therapy, as in the case with Mr. Martin. Others may want to take a break from therapy or quit altogether. While it will be best to try to notice shifts in the patient's connection with the provider right away, and to address their perceptions about how therapy is going, some-times the patient will not talk about his or her feelings (e.g., of distrust, hurt, disappointment) and will act on these feelings instead. This could manifest in the patient canceling sessions, not answering the door when the provider comes, or scheduling doctors' appointments at the same time as therapy. Re-establishing connection may require the provider to call and ask the patient how she/he felt about the past session or explore other feelings the patient has been having towards the provider and the therapy. In Mr. Martin's case, the MH provider asked him how he felt that the case manager had called 911.

If the patient does not respond to initial overtures from the MH provider, the provider will need to decide how many times to keep calling, and/or whether to make an unannounced home visit. Company policy may dictate how many times a provider will reach out with a patient, but it is also important for a provider to establish her or his personal threshold. It is important for the provider to consider whether the patient may be "no-showing" due to a practical issue, such as disconnected phone line or medical hospitalization, or whether the patient is deliberately trying to take a break or end therapy but is not assertive enough to say so outright. If the patient has clearly stated he or she does not want to continue, one request to discuss this can be warranted, but clear refusal of services must be respected. Additionally, it can be helpful for a provider to discuss in training or supervision how to handle medical emergencies, and when, if ever, to call 911 for a patient when the patient does not want 911 called.

Dealing with Countertransference

A number of common countertransference reactions may occur when doing psychotherapy in the home that are different from office-based care. Reactions may vary from strongly negative to positive. As with therapy in general, it is important for MH providers to be self-aware, to process feelings that arise (both internally and in supervision or consultation), and to avoid reacting based on feelings of countertransference unless clinically indicated.

As with concerns noted above related to "over functioning" for patients, when patients have numerous needs providers may feel pity for or the desire to "take care of" patients rather than working to empower them to develop the abilities and resources to take care of themselves. Providers may feel helpless when confronted with a patient who has a high level of need in multiple areas, such as having no family, having a disabling illness, and being impoverished. With the help of supervision, peer consultation, or mentorship, the provider can work to determine what can and cannot be done. MH providers may experience feelings of disgust (e.g., if a home smells of feces, or if there are bed bugs or cockroaches visible) and may need to give themselves permission to take care of themselves, such as requesting to open a window, meet on the porch, or make sessions shorter.

Feelings of frustration or anger are common when providers make significant efforts to go to a patient's home and the patient is not present for the session. This may be especially frustrating if the provider drives for an extra session or if the patient lives particularly far from the office. While reminder calls can assist with these difficulties, it still can happen. Processing this with a trusted colleague or discussing these issues with the patient can be helpful. Again, reviewing one's personal threshold can be helpful for tolerance of certain home-based experiences and behaviors.

On the other hand, the provider may feel a number of positive reactions. For example, getting to know the patient more personally, as the provider sees more intimate aspects of the patient and their home, could bring about a greater feeling of connection with the patient. The provider may feel particular affection for the patient, due to a sense of greater vulnerability of the patient's condition. The provider might also feel honored, or special, to be allowed into the patient's home.

Addressing Possible Crises or Safety Issues

It is important to be prepared to address crises from the very first session, and to voice any policies and procedures that may be helpful to the patient in setting the therapeutic frame. It is best to discuss with a supervisor, medical team, or consultant what to do if there is an indication of elder abuse, child abuse, self-neglect, a medical emergency, or suicidal or homicidal ideation or actions. See Chapter 6 for an in-depth discussion of crises and safety issues.

Summary

MH providers who see older adult patients in their homes can face numerous clinical, ethical, and practical decisions that can potentially affect the establishment and maintenance of therapeutic alliance. Seeing patients at home provides unique advantages to developing rapport, and there are several strategies that providers can use to maximize rapport. Home-based providers must be able to establish clear boundaries, and at times it may require extra effort to establish and maintain the professional therapeutic frame. As in Mrs. Johns' case, presented above, providers can use a patient's environment to develop rapport, remain flexible, and assert the need for privacy when family members are present. Conducting MH services in the home makes more visible the personal and practical needs of patients, and requires providers to consider a broader range of ethical and clinical decisions.

References

Maslow, A. H. (1943). A theory of human motivation. *Psychological Review, 50*, 370–396. doi:10.1037/h0054346.

Miller, W. R., & Rollnick, S. (1991). *Motivational interviewing: Preparing people to change addictive behavior*. New York, NY: Guilford Press.

Yang, J. A., Garis, J., Jackson, C., & McClure, R. (2009). Providing psychotherapy to older adults in home: Benefits, challenges, and decision-making guidelines. *Clinical Gerontologist, 32*, 333–346. doi:10.1080/07317110902896356.

Part 2
Practical Considerations

4 Managing the Home Setting and Mobile Office

Ann T. Landes and Carolyn T. Jackson

The day-to-day work life of a home care provider is both energizing and demanding. Because of the unique nature of the job, there are frequent opportunities to develop and refine specific skills and abilities. Flexibility, adaptability, communication, organizational, planning, and problem-solving skills are all necessary for working within the non-traditional settings of a patient's home and a mobile office. This chapter introduces practical strategies for working effectively and within the patient's home, from the initial phone contact to the in-home psychosocial assessment. The latter part of the chapter discusses the potential challenges of working within a mobile office, and suggests ways to improve one's efficiency, physical comfort, and psychological well-being.

Working in a Patient's Home

Preparing for the Home Visit

> After receiving a consult to provide mental health (MH) services for a 65-year-old woman with Amyotrophic Lateral Sclerosis, Dr. Rodriguez, the home care team's psychologist, calls the patient to schedule an appointment. Dr. Rodriguez successfully contacts the patient and after introductions and a short discussion about services, they agree to meet on Tuesday at 10 a.m. On the day of the appointment, Dr. Rodriguez arrives at the patient's home, but no one is there. Dr. Rodriguez calls the patient's cell number and is greeted by a caregiver. The caregiver expresses consternation that she did not know about the appointment and that Tuesdays are "out of the question" for home visits. The call ends abruptly with the caregiver saying, "Please, call back later."

The clinical intake provides critical information and serves as a guide for our work with patients. In home care, providers must do their own appointment scheduling, and the initial phone call is the first step of the intake process. During this interaction, MH providers typically introduce themselves to the patient, explain the reason for the call, describe the services being offered, and inquire about the patient's interest in services. Listening to, engaging with, and encouraging open communication with the patient helps gather information that will make the first home visit a positive and safe one. With the patient's permission, initial and subsequent contacts may involve and heavily rely upon the presence of a primary caregiver. Early in our home care careers, we realized that in order to be heartily invited into the life of the patient, we first had to gain the trust and cooperation of the caregiver. Hence, it is key to acknowledge the caregiver's contributions, express appreciation for their willingness to meet, and encourage them to be involved in at least the initial meeting.

The first phone contact focuses on communicating respect and the importance of the patient's autonomy throughout the therapeutic relationship. There are numerous other factors to consider while preparing for the first home visit. The initial call can assist with gathering information that aids in avoiding any "unpleasant surprises" in the home and sets the stage for open communication between the patient and MH provider. The provider might assess and prepare for the presence of unexpected individuals inside and outside of the home, be they human or animal. It is prudent to assess for specific health threats in the environment, like cigarette smoke, bed bugs, and other infectious agents (e.g., MRSA, flu).

Once identified, it is important to disclose the necessary precautions you will be taking during a home visit. Discuss the possible need for protective clothing (i.e., shoe covers, masks, gloves), so that the patient and family will not be left with uncomfortable assumptions or questions. Having knowledge about logistical considerations, such as the parking situation, how and where to enter a facility, and how to identify the home, will also help diminish stress-related surprises. See Chapter 6 for further discussion about managing specific safety concerns.

Every person has a stimulus value, or personal attributes that influence the way others perceive and engage with the MH provider. Examples of personal attributes include one's physical features, personality, communication style, and energy level. The stimulus value of the clinician within traditional MH settings is often taken for granted, as it is considered somewhat of a sterile or neutral territory. Unless one has the opportunity for a face-to-face meeting with the patient prior to the initial home visit, one will not know how the patient will respond to the provider's actual presence. In home care it is imperative that the clinician prepares the patient for your first home visit by appropriately disclosing any information that may trigger a strong emotional response from the patient. For example, the author (A.L.) had a patient with a diagnosis of post-traumatic stress disorder following trauma during the Vietnam War. She took the initiative and shared that she is of Asian descent

Table 4.1 Initial Contact Checklist

Task	Complete
Introduce yourself to the patient and family/caregiver(s)	□
Explain the reason for the call and the services being offered	□
Inquire about patient's interest; determine patient's ability to engage in services	□
Involve family/caregiver(s) as necessary, with the patient's permission	□
Discuss limits of confidentiality and obtain informed consent	□
Gather information about the home environment (e.g., health and safety concerns)	□
Discuss the possible need for protective clothing	□
Obtain information about parking, entrances, etc.	□
Schedule first home visit	□

and asked if the patient would be alright with the visit. The patient expressed appreciation for the information and replied that it would be fine. Prepping patients about what to expect with your arrival will reduce the likelihood of an unpleasant initial encounter. Table 4.1 provides a summary of the suggested steps discussed above.

Providing Treatment in the Home

Honoring the caregiver's request, Dr. Rodriguez waits until the next day and calls the patient. The caregiver answers and Dr. Rodriguez confirms it to be a good time to speak with her about scheduling a visit. The caregiver states that due to the patient's other appointments, fluctuating mental status, and schedule around aides providing personal care in the home, Monday mornings would be the best time to visit. Dr. Rodriguez reassures the caregiver that he would be glad to arrange his schedule to accommodate the request. On the day of the appointment, both the patient and caregiver are present. The caregiver offers Dr. Rodriguez a cup of coffee, but he politely declines, explaining that as the patient's MH provider he is focused on offering his professional expertise in helping the patient and the caregiver. Dr. Rodriguez provides information about the typical session length and inquires whether the patient could be situated in a more private space for each session. At the end of the session, Dr. Rodriguez talks with the patient about how the patient might spend the rest of the day. Dr. Rodriguez and the patient then collaboratively develop an action plan for addressing some of the identified life stressors and concerns. When the caregiver brings the calendar to schedule the next home visit, Dr. Rodriguez makes a point to express appreciation for how much caregivers must manage into order to attend to their loved one's health and well-being. As the caregiver walks Dr. Rodriguez to the door, she sighs and acknowledges feeling overwhelmed with trying to balance her own needs with those of her loved one. Dr. Rodriguez provides reflective listening and adds that he can be refer her to adjunct support services as well.

Considering the nature of many household environments, establishing therapeutic alliance while maintaining a confidential and therapeutic space can be one of the most unique components of providing effective behavioral treatment and support in this setting. Remember, we are working in the patient's private space, not the office. Thus, assisting the patient and/or caregiver(s) in developing ideas for preparing the home environment, or some part of it, to be conducive to psychotherapy should be a specific focus of initial interactions. Helping to ensure that a specific and private area in or around the home is set aside for the psychotherapy sessions can be as simple as reminding the patient that this time is for his or her well-being and that he or she is encouraged to honor that well-being by creating a section of the home that is quiet and free from the distraction of extraneous noise or others interrupting the confidential time for treatment and reflection. Consider how asking the patient "Do you mind if we turn down the radio? I want to be able to hear you better," or saying, "Perhaps you would prefer that we reschedule our visit for today. Since your aide is here, I want you to be able to spend all your personal care time with her" connotes care and concern around what the patient is sharing with you while honoring his or her privacy.

When providing care in this setting, MH providers should strive to bear in mind that providing psychotherapy in a person's home is perhaps the most distinctive setting in which one can be invited. Indeed, as the saying goes, "Home is where the heart is," and developing an appreciation for this truism is to value that no matter how big or small, clean or cluttered, this place is likely one of the patient's most essential personal sanctuaries.

Completing a Home-based Psychosocial Assessment

As discussed elsewhere in this text, psychosocial assessment of the patient's home, needs, expectations, receptivity to services, and readiness for change can begin even before the initial telephone contact is made. Indeed, there might be other service providers who have already been in the home, and their consultation reports and related records will often provide a rich source of information that helps us to begin to conceptualize the patient's behavioral strengths, challenges, and needs. Thus, it is likely to be well worth the effort to reach out to engage and collaborate with other entities involved in the psychosocial assessment process. Concurrently, MH providers will conduct their own psychosocial assessment to illuminate the collateral factors that might impact individual mental health and function. With this psychosocial assessment, home-based MH providers are specifically tasked with integrating data for an overall case conceptualization with the additional aim of determining specific domains that might warrant further expert evaluation and intervention. Many of these areas are immediately observable, while others will require a bit of time and discovery in the home.

Initially, one important area to be covered in the MH provider's psychosocial assessment is the home environment itself and the surrounding living circumstances, including the family or other social and therapeutic supports in place or lacking. It is important to explore how the environment and circumstances might impact the patient's daily and longer-term MH function and outlook. Other people involved in the patient's day-to-day living, home environment, or larger milieu might be of help or hindrance to the patient's mental well-being. When available, and when the patient allows, it can be helpful to interview and encourage support for the patient from these collateral sources. Sometimes the degree of involvement of other people in the patient's life directly relates to whether the patient is a viable candidate for various referral options. For instance, among the truly homebound (often older) patient population, individuals frequently have diminished access to means for managing basic activities of daily living (e.g., bathing) and instrumental activities of daily living (e.g., transportation). Including discussions related to these domains is important, as barriers related to fully engaging these tasks should be assessed and addressed to lessen their impact on the patient's ability to engage MH care and optimize well-being.

Another important component of the home-based psychosocial assessment involves evaluating the need for psychotropic medication. Given that patients receiving home care characteristically have diminished access to the specialty medical clinics, including psychiatry services, it can be helpful for MH providers to streamline engagement with the primary care providers already established with the patient to discuss prescriptions for psychotropic intervention. The MH provider can then provide continued in-home assessment and monitoring for any change in symptoms.

Including an assessment of the patient's attitudes, beliefs, traditions, and preferences in his or her individual religiosity and/or spirituality can also provide a wealth of information around the patient's biopsychosocial strengths and functioning. This can be as simple as enquiring about whether the patient was reared with any particular religious or spiritual beliefs, whether the patient currently engages any religious or spiritual practices, and whether the patient wishes to have these integrated into the current home-based MH treatment paradigm. Having the benefit of time with the patient in his or her home allows for candid observation of religious and/or spiritual tokens and literature that might be important to the patient's sense of well-being. Furthermore, by encouraging discussion around these conversation pieces during the psychosocial assessment, therapeutic rapport can be strengthened while providing an additional psychotherapeutic entry point for care.

All in all, consider that as home-based MH providers we have the dual opportunity of observing MH functioning in real time while often also serving as the first providers to discover additional therapeutic access areas that were not originally related to the primary consult question. Access to these types of clinical observations could be viewed as one of the most positive and patient-centered aspects of working in and managing MH care in the home, because as home care MH providers we inherently see far more real-time, *in vivo* data than would any other type of outpatient-based clinician. With this in mind, we should look to our psychosocial assessments to help clarify areas where we might help patients explore whether it could be of value for some of these to become the focus of treatment in and of themselves. For instance, consider how patient behaviors like tobacco use and hoarding of goods are naturally more observable in the home environment than in the clinic, and might be significant areas of malady and distress for the patient. At the same time, also consider how some matters that are present in this setting can be dangerous for not only the patient, but also the MH provider. Indeed, as discussed briefly above, tobacco smoke, soil, debris, and/or bed bugs or other infestations are all concerns that could negatively impact the health of anyone spending time in the home environment, including home-based clinical staff. Thus, inclusion of all of these factors in the psychosocial assessment can help other home-based staff better understand areas where the patient might need assistance and intervention and minimize harm to their own health and well-being.

The inherent goal of many home-based programs is to provide improved access to treatments, services, and supports that can in turn allow the patient to remain safe and independent in the home despite the comorbid maladies with which the individual is living. Applying some of the considerations outlined in this chapter can help us toward this goal, while also helping ensure the health and well-being of the treating MH provider.

Working Out of a Mobile Office

> Dr. Terri is a newly hired home care psychologist and is issued a car for her work. She is provided with a bag of first-aid-related items that needed to be stored for her potential use, but no other guidelines are provided. Dr. Terri sets out on her first day of home visits, armed with her notepad, cell phone, and daily calendar. As the day proceeds, Dr. Terri becomes stressed as she realizes that she does not have many items on hand that aid her in successfully performing her duties.

As compared to working within a traditional office setting, the mobile office environment takes mindful adaptation. Unexpected and daily events may result in minor inconveniences (i.e., interruptions in the schedule) or major upsets (i.e., safety issues). Taking the time to set up your mobile office and devising strategies for managing the unexpected can reduce job-related stress and give you more security of mind as you travel from site to site. This next section provides a convenient framework for addressing such concerns, which are divided into three categories: administrative, physical health and safety, and psychological well-being. As you read through this section, remember that there may be other creative solutions that will make your life on the road that much more enjoyable.

Administrative and Documentation Considerations

During her first several months as a home care provider, the author (A.L.) found that a significant source of stress was trying to adapt to her "new office" – a nondescript, government-issued compact car she named "Verna." She knew she would be spending many long hours with Verna, so she was determined to make this space as user-friendly as possible. Seeing Verna as an extension of herself and the quality services she strove to provide, her goal was to create an office space that reflected professionalism, stability, and reliability.

The provider can bring order to a mobile office space through an efficient document filing system. This is a little tricky when working in a vehicle, not only because of space issues, but also due to confidentiality. Guided by the rules of your organization and/or those that are Health Insurance Portability and Accountability Act-compliant, limiting and protecting the data that you transport is essential. Limit patient information to only critical data; generally, that would include addresses and phone numbers. We review patient medication lists and other pertinent treatment records prior to each visit. If you must carry the notes with you, de-identify the paperwork. In terms of transporting these, the most functional tool can be a portable locked file box kept in the trunk to store private documents. To ensure security, the file box can be purged of patient documents and locked in an office at the end of each workday.

Other key pieces of documentation that the provider might carry includes blank intake forms and MH screeners, which assess for issues such as depression, anxiety, sleep disorders, substance use, cognitive functioning, and suicidality, just to name a few. Patient educational materials and forms needed for psychiatric admission of patients can also be useful. For travel, the provider might employ the navigation device on one's phone, but if you know you will be travelling to a location with poor connectivity, you might also bring printed directions detailing routes to and from patients' homes as a backup.

There will be variation in the extent of clinical information other medical and social teammates will collect and document around the home visit, and every MH provider will likely follow an established local protocol regarding the extent of annotation he or she is expected to include regarding the MH provider psychosocial assessment. Despite this, consider documenting the information areas listed in Table 4.2 to capture some of the most important data.

Other necessary items include a cell phone with a charger and a business calendar that contains daily and weekly appointments. Within the auspices of working for the government or an agency, cash is generally not needed, but it may be prudent to have at least five dollars in change and small bills in the car to put air in the tires and pay for tolls, parking, etc. You may also carry mileage logs (or use a mobile app for this purpose) and an envelope for storing receipts. For those times when you need to reach your supervisor or colleagues, consider preprogramming them into your cell phone, and carrying a one-page listing of all key personnel, as well as emergency numbers for assistance in the event of a car breakdown and accident. (If

Table 4.2 Patient Record Documentation

Information Area	Documented
Location of encounter	☐
Session duration	☐
Diagnoses based on *DSM 5*	☐
Other (i.e., medical) diagnoses	☐
Presentation and mental status	☐
Risk factors including suicidal and homicidal ideation	☐
Current home living environment and circumstances	☐
Additional treatment issues (e.g., tobacco use)	☐
Medical history, including chief complaint	☐

you are driving a fleet car, you will likely be instructed to call a specific number for roadside assistance.) And, of course, make sure that there are writing utensils, paper, paperclips, and tape on hand.

An additional consideration is how you will manage the technology you bring into the home or those technologies that are already present in this setting. While you can refer to Chapter 15 for additional recommendations and discussion around clinical video teleconferencing and telehealth in the provision of care in the home, consider how you will interface with your organization (or personal) cell phone or smartphone while providing psychotherapeutic services in this setting. Just as you might ask the patient to turn down the television or radio during the visit, you should consider silencing your own technology for the session time. Of course, if you do have service area coverage, it is good to be able to receive emergency clinical alerts that can be addressed following your time with the current patient, and it is also essential to be able to receive emergency administrative, weather, and/or disaster alerts from your agency while you are in the field.

Unlike outpatient work, providers commonly bring and use smartphones in the home during the session. You will want to ensure that you are not interacting with your technology in the home unless it is with the intention of serving the patient's needs. For instance, you might use your smartphone to remotely access information in the patient's medical record, check your calendar to schedule the patient's next home visit, or review scientific literature regarding the patient's condition(s). Policymakers within and across organizations continue to debate the potential benefits and drawbacks of patients using their own technology and devices during the home-based session to produce their own footage and/or other documentation of the interaction. It is best to refer to your local institutional directives for guidance around how to address a patient's wish to use his or her own instruments, monitors, or other recording devices during your home visit.

Managing Your Own Personal Comfort

Half-way through the day the weather becomes unseasonably rainy, with sleet. Dr. Terri did not expect these conditions, and hence did not bring a raincoat. She feels relieved that she has an umbrella in the car. However, Dr. Terri soon learns that the windshield wiper blades are in need of replacement as they are failing to clean the windshield appropriately, leaving her with low visibility. Dr. Terri wants to stop and purchase new blades, but she is in a rural setting and does not know the area.

Maintaining your own physical comfort both in the home and on the road can easily be overlooked or regarded as unimportant as you become more efficient on the job. When one considers all that needs to be accomplished for even a single visit, it becomes obvious why attending to your own self-care (and the care of your vehicle) is critical to our short- and long-term job survival.

Environmental set-up may be the easiest factor to prepare and manage. Being both our mode of transportation and office, the vehicle needs to be cared for so that it remains reliable and safe. Scheduled tune-ups are essential, along with regular brake servicing, oil changes, tire checks, windshield wiper replacement and fluid refills, and inspection of exterior lights to be sure they are working properly. Know your vehicle and be aware of any signs that indicate the need for service. Purchasing a car emergency kit and first aid supplies for the vehicle is highly recommended. These suggestions apply regardless if it is a personal car or part of a fleet. The only difference that may arise is that fleet service cars are scheduled for maintenance by your company, with you being responsible for taking the car in for service when notified.

Accommodating for seasonal changes and needs is another important consideration. For example, during the warmer months, have items in the car like a sunhat, cotton scarf and/or long-sleeved shirt to provide extra protection from the sun, while a change of shoes or an extra sweater can be useful to have in the car during the winter. Sunglasses and an umbrella are often useful, regardless of the season. Carrying items like hand sanitizer; baby wipes; sunscreen; lip balm; lotions and ointments for dry, cracked hands and fingers; allergy and cold medicines; lozenges; aspirin; eye drops; and saline nose spray can all be helpful when far from the comforts of an outpatient office or home.

Depending on the distances the provider is required to drive, he or she may experience strain from driving. Like the car, our bodies experience wear, such as in the lower back from sitting for long periods of time and the neck and shoulders from holding a steering wheel, and eye strain from bright light. To mitigate these effects, consider employing a seat cushion and lumbar support, integrate stretches throughout the day, and don appropriate eye wear. You might also consult with an ergonomics professional to adjust your seat and mirrors to minimize strain.

In the same vein we must consider a rudimental creature comfort: a bathroom. At times, the simple task of attending to bodily functions truly strengthens one's executive functioning skills! Be it an urban or rural setting, locating a (clean and safe) public restroom – anywhere near the patient's home – proves challenging. Planning your route each day to include essential pit stops is critical. Asking co-workers to disclose their "secret locations" is also quite helpful. Navigation apps can be used to pinpoint potential places to stop. While some of the most obvious places, like gas stations, grocery stores, pharmacies, fast food restaurants, and mini-marts, are generally safe bets, there are instances when access to a bathroom is denied. With a little ingenuity, a desperate situation can be transformed to a relieving one. Consider, for instance, using the facilities in a public library, hospital, or community park. Porta-potties are also an option, as well as a portable urinal. A co-worker once disclosed that something as simple as a large jar can make a difference between a good and bad day. One more pertinent suggestion: When entering an establishment to use the facilities, be interpersonally appropriate and if need be, purchase an item. This will pave the way for positive interactions at businesses you may need to return to in the future.

Because the job entails extensive travelling, not being in an office setting, and a solitary experience, some may find it difficult to define what is appropriate work attire. There are several useful questions when determining what to wear as a home care provider. Are you able to perform your job safely (for the patient and self) with the chosen apparel and accessories? On a similar note, are you able to freely move about, quickly if needed, without being harmed (e.g., falling, choked) or hampered from ill-chosen garments, footwear, etc.? Does your professional attire match the environment, not only with regard to weather, but socioeconomic, cultural, and religious norms of the patient's home and surrounding neighborhood? Are they machine-washable or will you be incurring large dry-cleaning bills? If the answer to any of these questions leaves you in doubt about your ability to function in a healthy and safe manner, it may be best to reconsider the chosen garments. See Chapter 3 for more discussion on the impact of professional attire on developing the therapeutic relationship.

Psychological Well-Being

It is toward the end of the day and Dr. Terri is scheduled to complete an initial assessment with Mr. Lang, a 55-year-old man. Dr. Terri relies on her GPS system to get her to patients' homes, but due to the rural nature of this particular area her GPS system fails to provide the exact location. Dr. Terri calls the patient three times to verify directions, but no one answers. After about 30 minutes of driving and searching, she finally pulls into what she hopes is Mr. Lang's driveway. Upon parking the car in front of the home, Dr. Terri is greeted on the lawn by a man who appears confused and either unwilling or unable to respond to her questions. Dr. Terri returns to her car, feeling uncertain about what to do or who to call. She is physically, emotionally, and psychologically exhausted.

The road is a beautiful place, filled with expectations and natural wonder, challenging us on many different levels. We've discussed the importance of establishing an efficient and functional mobile office, and addressed ways to increase physical health and safety. This section will highlight one area that is possibly the most critical of the three: our psychological well-being.

Psychological well-being is a subjective concept that encompasses feelings of mastery, contentment, and autonomy; a sense of meaning and purpose; and positive relations with others. As a home care provider, your psychological well-being may be challenged daily due to the solitary nature of the job. Unless you travel as a team, time on the road can feel isolating. You no longer have the convenience of walking down a hallway to discuss, process, and consult with colleagues about the daily consequential and not-so-consequential events. Opportunities to attend meetings and participate within team settings are limited. Navigating the daily demands of the job – alone – can lead to a build-up of stress and eventual burnout.

The good news is that it is possible to create a network of support to bolster your psychological well-being. For instance, to increase a sense of community, and for safety reasons, let office staff know the places you are scheduled to be throughout the day and when to expect you back at the office. At least once a week, set an appointment with a colleague for either an in-person or phone meeting to discuss work-related concerns, seek consultation, or simply process a difficult case. For emergent issues, be astute about the departmental process for reaching someone, be it your supervisor for clinical concerns or a roadside assistance company for car-related items.

Not only can the feeling of being disconnected from a support network impact your work, but physical, emotional, and psychological fatigue are also occupational hazards within the home care field. They cause stress and burnout, which in turn can result in decreased effectiveness and increased absenteeism from the job. Hence, it is imperative that during the work day there is time set aside for physical stretching (e.g., create reminders about stretching throughout the day), nourishment and relaxation of our bodies and soul (e.g., tune in to calming music, dedicate time to eat a healthy meal), social connectedness (i.e., become a mentor or a mentee), and stimulation of our minds (i.e., listen to an educational program, learn a new language). These activities can occur practically anywhere – a gas station, in the car, or even at a library. Just remember to be cautious about where and when you decide to stop.

As highlighted in this chapter, managing the home setting as a home care provider can be both thorny and gratifying. If new and seasoned MH providers alike can review and apply some of the strategies outlined here, each encounter with patients can result in positive behavioral health outcomes for the patient and a sense of professional effectiveness for the

MH provider. All providers involved in home care encounters have the potential to develop means for successfully navigating nearly any challenge that arises in this setting, and in doing so can provide increased treatment access for patients, clearing the way for their pursuit of the best quality of life they can possibly experience.

5 A Private-Practice Model of Providing Mental Health Services for Older Adults

Perspectives of a Practicing Provider

Maureen E. Sweeney

Providing home-based mental healthcare is about social justice. It is about providers making a reasonable accommodation about where the service is rendered to enable seniors to obtain access to healthcare that otherwise would not be obtainable.

Anonymous

Mrs. Kurkawa is a 66-year-old retired, widowed, Japanese American woman. She called last week to request an appointment, stating, "I just need to talk to someone, I am having a lot of problems in my life right now. Even I know I need help." She explains that she has Medicare insurance with the AARP supplemental plan. She lives alone in a condominium retirement community within a few miles of my business office. I explain that I specialize in geriatric psychology and that I travel to all of my patients to provide care because many of them no longer drive and have difficulty getting to medical appointments. She replies,

> Are you kidding me? That is perfect. I still drive, but my kids want me to stop. I don't get around as much as I used to. If the only way to get into a building is to go up steps, I just don't go in anymore.

When asked, Mrs. Kurkawa explains that she was at the doctor's office last week and that her health is "pretty good." She explains that she is not suicidal, although her doctor asked because he said he noticed that she is more depressed than she has been. Mrs. Kurkawa and I schedule an appointment for the following week. I explain to her that I have a web page with my picture, so she can see what I look like before I arrive at her apartment for the appointment next week. She explains that she already saw the picture and web page when she was on the computer looking for someone to talk to. She said that I had a lot of good information on the web page about what I do, and that is why she called me.

At the initial appointment, Mrs. Kurkawa says she desperately misses her husband of 45 years who died of cancer two years ago. She begins to cry as she explains that she called because her youngest daughter is now going through cancer treatments and things are not going well. Mrs. Kurkawa explains that her daughter has four children, and that her marriage and family are falling apart because of the illness. She begins to sob as she reports that she is trying to do all she can to help, but that two weeks ago her son-in-law lost his temper and yelled that she needed to leave their house because she was "not helping, only making things worse."

And so the course of cognitive-behavioral therapy for adjustment disorder with symptoms of depression begins. The treatment goals are: (1) to reduce symptoms of depression, (2) to increase coping skills, (3) to further develop strategies on how to support her daughter and younger grandchildren during their time of stress (without agitating the son-in-law), (4) to increase knowledge and coping related to normal aging processes (i.e., decline in ability to get around, the question of when to stop driving), and (5) to provide support for the ongoing grieving process related to the loss of her husband, and the grieving process related to the loss of the good health of her daughter.

After the first session, Mrs. Kurkawa stated that she really thinks the counseling will help her and that she looks forward to the next visit. Over the next two months, Mrs. Kurkawa learns new coping strategies related to her symptoms of depression and related to the stressors in her life. Even as the health of her daughter continues to be a concern, Mrs. Kurkawa demonstrates a decrease in her symptoms of depression. In fact, she now gives my card to several of her friends and tells her doctor about how counseling really works. Her doctor then asks her to relay a message to her therapist after a follow-up medical appointment. The message indicates that he can see that the mental health (MH) treatment is helping Mrs. Kurkawa very much. He has never heard of an MH provider delivering the care to older adults in the home, and that he thinks this is a needed service for older adults. In fact, he knows of a few older adults whom he thinks could benefit from counseling in the home, and I am invited to call the doctor if the therapist has any open appointment slots for new clients.

Over the past 15 years, I have developed, implemented, and continue to grow a private-practice model of delivering MH services to older adults at home. At the start, I ventured out on this practice development project armed with only my professional license in Psychology, and a Certificate of Completion of a Post-Doctoral Fellowship in Geriatric Psychology. This chapter highlights some basic considerations of providing home care as a private-practice provider.

The purpose of this chapter is to discuss the development of a private-practice model of MH services to older adults at home. When delivering home-based MH services to older adults, most aspects of the care remain the same as care provided in the office. However, there are important practice concerns that are unique to delivering home-based services that need to be addressed. These include: (1) knowledge about how Medicare and Medicaid programs fund and impact (directly and indirectly) how MH care can be provided to older adults at home; (2) ensuring that the care is appropriate, competent, effective, ethical, and safe to provide in the home; and (3) understanding how providing home care influences marketing, charting, and billing policy and procedures.

Developing a Private Practice

The first step in setting up a home care practice was to write a comprehensive business plan. This involved spending a couple of hundred dollars to buy the bestselling business plan software program on the market at the time. It continues to be a top-selling program for any small business startup and was perfect for my use in setting up my sole practice psychology business. Some of the most important aspects of working as a psychologist include understanding and implementing business concepts that graduate school does not teach.

When identifying a business plan, it was necessary to clearly define my business, identify earning goals, write a mission statement, and identify factors key to the success of the business. The program instructed me on how to conduct a market analysis. For example, I was able to look up demographic information for my town and county and state regarding the total number of the general population and what percent of the population is over age 65. Then I was able to compare that to the national average. I was able to confirm that both the county and state where I live have a higher-than-the-national-average number of residents who are older than age 65, and the numbers are expected to grow in the decades ahead. Also, the Medicare fees paid for behavioral health services can be looked up by geographic area on the Center for Medicare Services website. Finally, and most importantly, the software program was able to help me to develop and implement a marketing strategy on how to connect with the clients to provide the service. Within one week, I had a business plan.

The second step to starting my practice was to find a part-time job as a psychologist to generate an income while I developed my own practice. Generally, it takes about three years to get a new business from the ground up to generating a profit. I found that it took three years before I was able to leave the part-time job and launch into full-time private practice.

Right now, I am credentialed and on-staff at a local hospital system that includes several short-term rehabilitation units, several long-term-care skilled nursing units, and an independent living housing unit.

I dedicate about two days a week to the hospital system, and three days a week to home care. All clinical care I provide is within 10 miles of my office. I schedule home visits by day of the week and by county. I travel to three different counties in the state where I live. I schedule between three and eight appointments per day, for an average of 25 to 30 appointments per week. I travel on average for 15 minutes between appointments. I live in a densely populated geographic area with extensive non-congested highways that allow me to travel within a county with more ease than may be possible in other areas of the country.

I have several referral sources, and I continue to develop new referral sources daily. For instance, other healthcare providers at the hospital system observe the quality and helpfulness of my work and then ask to refer more patients who live within the community. Often, I will encounter nurses from nursing agencies providing care at the same home and the nurses will ask about my services and request if they can provide my name to others who they think could benefit from the home-based MH services. I have a comprehensive website that includes my picture and a description of the services I provide, as well as my curriculum vitae (CV). Because providing behavioral health services in the home is new and innovative, I provide more information about my practice and about myself than most providers would feel is necessary. I do this because I recognize that older adults and their family members can be expected to be leery about psychological care being provided in the home that is not affiliated with the nursing agencies that most members of the community are familiar with.

I have had affiliation with several long-term care (LTC) facilities in the area since starting my practice. Except for the hospital affiliation, business relationships and referral streams can ebb and flow for reasons unrelated to my practice and the care I provide. For example, a facility administrator may contact me about meeting to discuss my providing care to residents in the building, and the successful relationship continues if that administrator continues to work at the facility. The ebb and flow of facility affiliation is just part of the business of working within the LTC system.

Because I am the only psychology provider in the area who renders the care that I provide, my schedule remains at about 95 percent full. I generally turn away two appointments for every one new appointment that I can accommodate into my schedule each week. Based on my experience over the past 15 years, and census data, there is growing demand for behavioral health care services provided to older adults at the home.

The Impact of Medicare and Medicaid Programs

The first question that needs to be answered when talking about any healthcare service program is, "How will the bill for service be paid?" The answer to this question is the same for every patient, whether MH services are provided to older adults in the home or in the office.

Currently, the Medicare insurance plan will pay for the Psychological Evaluation (90791) and Psychotherapy Follow-Up Visit (90832, 90834, 90837). How the bill will be paid is the easy question to answer. At times, the much more difficult questions to answer are: (1) Which type of Medicare plan does the prospective client have? (2) Is there a co-payment required at the time of the service? and (3) If yes, what is the amount of co-payment that is due? I have observed that only about 20 percent of referred older adults who use a Medicare HMO (health maintenance organization) plan will schedule an appointment with me after I indicate they are required to pay a $40 co-pay for each appointment. This is contrasted with the nearly 100 percent scheduling affirmation of the older adults who use Original Medicare insurance with a supplemental plan and who are informed that there is not an out-of-pocket expense for the psychology services provided.

Most older adults have their insurance card near at hand when calling to schedule the first appointment. The caller can report the information printed on the card that the MH provider can then use to confirm the type of Medicare plan and to determine if a co-payment is required. It is important to confirm the insurance information and to inform the patient of any out-of-pocket expenses for the service before scheduling the first appointment. It can be inconvenient for the provider to arrive at the patient's home for the first appointment only to learn that the patient did not know they would be required to pay anything for the service, and they want to cancel the appointment because they cannot afford the co-payment.

Although most people probably hear the words "Medicare" and "Medicaid" at least once a week during a news broadcast, many people do not know the difference between these two critically important funding programs. Table 5.1 lists some of the basic differences between Medicare and Medicaid and highlights the most important aspects of these programs as they relate to older adults and MH services provided in the home.

The primary difference between Medicare and Medicaid is the population each program serves. Medicare is a health insurance plan for older adults and the disabled, while Medicaid provides mostly non-medical and social programs for the economically disadvantaged of all ages. Notably, Medicare health insurance is determined by age or disability, not whether someone is retired or still working.

When MH services are provided to older adults in the home, services are billed through Medicare Part B, not through the Medicare Home Health program. The Medicare Home Health program provides a bundled payment to a home health agency to supply medical care that traditionally would be provided in a doctor's office or a hospital to the patient at home. The patient must qualify to receive services through the Medicare Home Health program. MH services are not covered under the program.

Table 5.1 Basic Differences between Medicare and Medicaid

	Medicare	Medicaid
What is it?	Health insurance	Mostly non-medical social service programs for the financially eligible
Types of plans	There are three types of plans: 1. *Original Medicare*: usually with a Medigap supplemental plan, covers 100 percent of the Medicare maximum allowed amount for MH services 2. *Medicare PPO*: covers less than the Medicare maximum allowed amount for MH services *and* the client must pay a $10–$40 co-pay per visit for MH services 3. *Medicare HMO*: covers less than the Medicare maximum allowed amount for MH services *and* the client must pay at least a $40 co-pay per visit for MH services	If someone is dual-eligible, sometimes the state Medicaid plan will help pay the Medicare co-payment. Usually the Medicare provider must also be enrolled as a Medicaid provider to receive the Medicaid co-payment benefit that the client may be eligible to receive
Who qualifies?	American citizens aged 65 and older or those that have received Social Security Disability Benefits for more than two years	Any person of qualifying economic status
Types of programs	*Medicare Part A*: pays hospital benefits *Medicare Part B*: pays doctor's visits provided in the office or in the home *Medicare Part D*: prescription benefits *Medicare Home Health Care Program*: this pays for after-hospital-stay follow-up at home for a few weeks (it does *not* pay for MH care in the home)	There are many types of programs for all age groups. The most important program for older adults is the Medicaid nursing home waiver program – this pays for ongoing non-medical home care services such as help with dressing and bathing, and for meals to the poor who would need nursing home care if the non-medical home care services were not provided
Is this the same in every state?	Original Medicare is the same in every state The PPOs (preferred provider organizations) and HMOs will be different from state to state	Not at all. In higher-tax areas, there are usually more Medicaid programs available. There can be significant differences in Medicaid programs from state to state

As mentioned above, most older adults referred to me report that they cannot afford the $40 co-pay and they make too much money to qualify for Medicaid assistance with paying the Medicare HMO co-pay. These prospective patients either decline the needed MH services, or they will state that due to the co-pay requirement that they can only attend appointments once a month rather than the needed weekly visits. In other instances, families may insist on the need for the older adult to receive needed MH services in the home, and a family member will contract with the provider to pay the weekly co-pay for MH services. The HMO co-payment can be a significant barrier to obtaining behavioral health care for the older adults who choose this type of Medicare insurance plan.

There are several strategies to handle this problem. First, the provider can ask the patient or family member to help to cover the cost. Second, the provider can make a referral to a social worker to determine whether the patient qualifies for Medicaid assistance with covering the co-pay. Also, finally referring the patient to the Area Agencies on Aging can help the patient evaluate if choosing a different Medicare plan at the open enrollment window in the fall will help them to obtain access to specialists without an additional out-of-pocket cost. Patients and their families need education about choosing the best Medicare plan based on the care needs of the older adult.

In summary, it is important to confirm the insurance of the prospective patient and discuss any out-of-pocket co-payment that is due at the time of service before the first appointment is scheduled. It is necessary to understand that the patient may be receiving concurrent services in the home under the Medicare Home Health Services program (due to a recent hospitalization). Similarly, it is important to understand that the patient may be receiving non-medical services (i.e. help with bathing, dressing, housekeeping) at home under the Medicaid nursing home waiver program. This program allows qualifying older adults to receive non-medical care in the home, and the psychology services provided in the home are billed by the provider under the Medicare Part B insurance plan.

Of note, there is a special billing issue related to Medicare when the MH service is provided to the older adult at home. This service is billed under the Location of Service (LOC) Code of Professional Office (location code 11) rather than LOC of Patient's Home (location code 12). The Professional Office code is used because the MH services are provided by an independent healthcare provider as an outpatient medical appointment rather than as part of a bundled payment service provided by a home health services agency. MH services are excluded for payment under bundled payment services provided by home health service agencies that are paid by both Medicare and Medicaid funding programs. This is the primary reason that home health service agencies do not hire MH providers to provide services as part of the home health agency's continuum of care. Working directly in the field, I advocate that the behavioral health services continue to be provided as part of the Medicare Part B plan. One might argue that it would improve the provision of behavioral health services.

A Non-traditional MH Service Delivery Model

Because providing MH services to older adults in the home is a non-traditional service delivery concept, special attention must be given to ensure that the care is appropriate, competent, effective, ethical, and safe to provide the care in the home. Before an MH provider can professionally render MH services to older adults in the home, the private-practice provider must develop a clear definition of what their scope of practice entails when providing the care in the home. For example, I am an MH-trained sole practitioner who travels into the community alone. Therefore, I do not provide any type of crisis intervention service within my practice. However, there exists a community clinic that provides a mobile crisis care geriatric MH assessment team that is able to competently and safely provide crisis geriatric home-based MH assessment because the clinic can send out a team of providers to conduct the assessment, including a registered nurse, a social worker, and an MH provider. Because I only see patients under Medicare, I follow Medicare policies and procedures related to Psychological Evaluation and Psychotherapy Follow-up. As a result, when providing care to a client in the community when the diagnosis of the client is major neurocognitive disorder (dementia), I am sure to evaluate and document at each session that the client has the cognitive capacity to benefit from the psychotherapy follow-up service.

The Telephone Screening Questionnaire I use allows me to quickly determine whether the service needs of the prospective client match up with my defined scope of practice. I find this to be the single most important tool that I use in my practice to ensure that the care I provide is appropriate, competent, effective, ethical, and safe. See Table 5.2 for examples of many of the questions that the prospective client is asked before the first appointment is scheduled.

The questionnaire is a tool that is used to determine if the prospective client is appropriate to schedule an appointment with. If the prospective client is eligible; then the Initial Psychological Evaluation is scheduled at the end of the phone call. If scheduling an appointment with me is not appropriate for the prospective client, I clearly explain the reason why to the person on the phone. Then, I provide suggestions about where they may be able to find the service they are seeking. Having a list of viable services or options promotes ethical and quality service.

When administering the questionnaire, there is a conversational flow to obtaining the answers to the questions. Often the callers will spontaneously provide much of the pertinent information without my having to ask most of the questions. If scheduling an appointment with me is not appropriate, the call usually takes about three to five minutes. If the prospective client is eligible to schedule an appointment, I will spend more time verifying the insurance plan and beginning to collect background information that will be applied during the Initial Psychological

Table 5.2 The Telephone Screening Questionnaire

Question	Response
How old are you?	
What is your address?	
I provide the care in the home. Is that alright with you?	
How did you hear about me?	
What is your insurance plan?	
Can I confirm your insurance with you?	
If there is a co-pay for each visit, are you agreeable to making the payment?	
How would you like me to help you?	
Who do you live with?	
Is there a location in the home where we can have a private conversation during the appointment?	
If you have psychiatric medications, who prescribes them for you?	
When was the last appointment you had with your medical doctor?	
Are you in medical or psychiatric crisis?	
Are you suicidal? *(Complete phone assessment as appropriate)*	
Are you primarily looking for memory care services?	
Have you left a hospital or nursing home against medical advice in the past 30 days?	

Evaluation. This extended telephone conversation also allows for an opportunity to support the development of a positive therapeutic alliance. In this situation, calls last about 15 to 20 minutes. Consequently, when I arrive for the first appointment the client already has some sense of who I am and how I provide care.

The Community and Referral Sources

Often, the public, other service providers, and even the PPO and HMO insurance plans can hold incorrect ideas about homecare. It is important to explain often the psychotherapy services one provides. It has been my experience that the public can view the home-based MH services as a Medicare-insurance-paid in-home dementia care activity program. There have been times when insurance company staff would call to request that I provide in-home crisis intervention care in order to stave off a need for psychiatric hospitalization. In addition, a provider might discontinue care with an older adult when it becomes apparent that the older adult only requested the MH services for themselves at home in an attempt to obtain MH support for a much younger adult family member who needed MH services and was refusing to seek those services in the community. Resourceful? Yes. Appropriate? No.

In conclusion, because providing MH services to older adults in the home is a non-traditional private service delivery model, it is essential that the MH provider develop a clear definition of the scope of practice. Once a clear scope of practice is defined, then a personalized Telephone Screening Questionnaire can be developed that allows for a quick determination of whether the service needs of a prospective client match with the scope of practice of the MH provider.

Administrative Considerations: Marketing, Charting, and Billing Procedures

There are important administrative considerations when providing MH services to older adults at home. Because this is a newer service model, it can be helpful to develop a web page or other online presence that includes a detailed description of the scope of practice and services provided. It can be useful to include a current picture of oneself so that new patients can know what the provider looks like when she arrives at their door for the first appointment. The provider might also include a CV on the web page. Ordinarily, a detailed CV may not be necessary on an MH practice web page. Because providing MH services to older adults at home is less familiar to others, I have found that other providers, especially geriatric providers working in the community, use my web page to learn more about the services that I offer, and perhaps more importantly to ensure that the healthcare service provider utilizes a professional, competent, ethical, and safe service delivery model.

All documentation of home care services is the same as care provided in an office. In fact, many MH providers who render services to older adults in the home also have a professional office where services are provided to other clients. As an exclusive home care provider, I have formally established a professional business office for my practice within my home. I do not provide any health-care services within my home, but I do incorporate a formal business office as part of the important administrative aspects of a model of care that provides the services at the location of the patients. Over the years, I have developed partnerships and consulting staff privileges with a number of LTC facilities located within the community. Sometimes I can follow my patients from the home setting to the LTC setting. The continuity of care is seamless when my patient is admitted to an LTC where I provide care.

Summary

Providing MH services to older adults at home is a relatively new, innovative, non-traditional, and in-demand service delivery model. Just like office-based work, the same ethical and other practice principles apply. There are three significant aspects specific to providing mental care to older adults at home that require the attention of the provider. The first practice issue is developing a strong understanding of how the Medicare and Medicaid programs fund and influence how care is provided in the home. As regulations and laws evolve and change, it is important to seek out resources to continue to educate oneself about these changes. It can be helpful to receive Medicare provider emails about upcoming changes in the Medicare program, and through geropsychology organizations and listservs. The second practice issue is the concern about the need to define one's scope of practice. This will allow the provider to develop a Telephone Screening Questionnaire that can be used as a tool to quickly determine if the MH needs of the prospective patient match with the services that the provider renders. Finally, it is important to understand how providing the care in the home influences marketing strategies, charting, and Medicare billing policies and procedures.

6 Managing Safety Concerns in Home Care

Danielle L. Terry and Brian Zuzelo

> Outpatient work is like swimming in an aquarium. Home-based work is like swimming in an ocean.
>
> Anonymous

Mrs. Kapuscinski was a 94-year-old, white, widowed woman who lived in a two-story colonial home on a quiet street. Mrs. Kapuscinski's nurse practitioner had asked the team psychologist, Dr. Hendrik, to meet with Mrs. Kapuscinski after the medical team noticed cognitive concerns and increasing confusion. On two recent occasions Mrs. Kapuscinski had called the police late at night, believing that a man was living in the upstairs of her home. Mrs. Kapuscinski was frail, and her family was involved, but on an "as-needed" basis. Dr. Hendrik had assisted with a psychological assessment and provided safety recommendations to the team. Following her recommendations, Mrs. Kapuscinski began receiving daily home health aide support and meal preparation. Her family began to assist with setting up a medication tray, and they moved her to the first floor of her house, so she could avoid the stairs. Dr. Hendrik planned to visit Mrs. Kapuscinski on a monthly basis to assist with monitoring of safety concerns.

During her fourth visit, Dr. Hendrik pulled into Mrs. Kapuscinski's driveway on a hot summer afternoon and found Mrs. Kapuscinski slumped in a woven aluminum lawn chair, eyes closed. Dr. Hendrik noticed that Mrs. Kapuscinski was positioned in the shade of a maple tree, but with the shifting daylight, nearly half of her was exposed to the sun. She had a mostly filled take-out beverage tilted on the ground next to her, and several bandages were wrapped around her arms and legs. Dark red stains were visible through the bandages, and a few small rivulets of blood soaked a trail down her bright white slacks.

The home care environment subjects the provider to a variety of risks and challenges not found within the more sterile clinical environment. At times, those challenges will be anticipated, and can be addressed proactively. As with the case above, providers may arrive and realize that they must respond to a more emergent situation. There are a variety of factors that home care MH providers must consider regarding their own safety. Managing the weather, pets, transportation, and weapons adds a complexity to care that can be terrifying at worst, and invigorating at its best. The provider must negotiate clinical practice needs and one's own intuition about personal safety. This chapter highlights guiding principles to consider prior to and while providing home care, and specific tips and tricks to manage common safety obstacles on the job.

Guiding Principles

Whether you are an individual who is working within a team or work by yourself, there are several precautions you can take to ensure your own safety. Safety strategies can be divided into proactive and reactive, or things that you do prior to leaving for your destination and what you might do to manage difficult and unexpected situations once you are there.

Being Prepared (Before You Go)

Know Your Referral Source

Many patients in home care are not self-referred, or even seeking psychological services. They may have limited to no experience with therapy and assessment. And every encounter begins with a referral point. Although the nature and the source of the referral can differ by setting, it is important to know who is sending you the referral, and how familiar he or she may be with the nature of home care. Certain referral sources have the best intentions when initiating psychology services. Yet they may not always realize the fact that the nature of the visit may be more emotionally charged than visits from other disciplines and that some household members may not be receptive to the service. Often, providers who are unfamiliar with home care may disregard safety concerns, as they are not relevant to the outpatient setting. They may see home care as a "catch all," or even a last-ditch effort to help a patient who is not showing up to outpatient care. If this is the case, the primary question to the referral source may be "What do you think home care will add to this patient's healthcare? What is it that is keeping the patient from coming to outpatient care?" In addition, it may be useful to directly inquire about safety issues or concerns the referral source may have about the patient or his or her home situation.

For providers who receive regular referrals from the same source, it can be useful to provide education and review with that source what constitutes an appropriate referral, and note any specific concerns to look for. For example, it can be helpful to identify individuals who have previously been incarcerated for sexual or violent crimes, who are actively using recreational drugs, or who have a history of becoming aggressive with providers prior to accepting a referral. It is important that the MH provider carefully consider the interpersonal dynamics between a referral source and the patients they refer. Some referrals may be made to mitigate feelings they have about the patient, but this may not be what the patient really wants or needs.

Examine Past Medical Records

If you have the privilege of using an electronic health record, or have access to past medical records, there are several things to consider when screening for safety issues. First, there may be specific safety issues flagged within the chart. There may be specific medical conditions like MRSA or other infections that you need to protect yourself from. Suicide risk assessments or past violent behavior may be flagged or noted on the face sheet of the chart. Second, you may be able to mine the medical data for more information. Previous social work assessments, occupational therapy assessments or other medical notes may provide clues to social history, drug use, or the patient's home setting. Checking laboratory results or drug and alcohol use screens, or examining chief complaints for emergency room visits, may yield no information, but may also shed light on patterns that suggest safety concerns. You will also be far more prepared to manage the challenges of working with patients with delirium or dementia as well. Aggressive or hyper-sexual behavior can be put into context more easily with a clear understanding of the patient's medical history.

Use Your Team

MH providers may work within a team, and/or have contacts within the community. Often, in settings like home-based primary care, a nurse or other individual may have already met the patient at his or her home. Keeping an open line of communication and briefly asking whether there are any specific concerns prior to initiating a visit may easily help one detect any issues. It may be useful to ask others who have visited the patient about anything they noticed regarding the home situation, or concerns about weapons or irregular behavior, or concerns related to where the patient lives. Simply asking about safety concerns may not be adequate, as team members from different disciplines and backgrounds may not notice or identify specific behaviors or situations as potentially risky. Of course, it is important to comply with confidentiality restrictions with those individuals that may not be affiliated with your organization, but it is also acceptable to ask about environmental concerns in a specific area of town or an apartment complex prior to going there.

Many providers may consider doing joint visits with other team members, particularly for patients who have a history of inappropriate sexual behavior or violence, or if there is a known family member with similar difficulties. Conducting a joint visit with a colleague who has an established relationship with the patient may have the downside of restricting the patient's openness in therapy, but may also have the effect of curbing inappropriate behavior or providing "strength in numbers." Conversely, a joint visit may help build on positive rapport developed with other providers and send a message of unity among the teams about certain policies related to safety. Joint visits may be particularly helpful for patients who struggle with reactive behavior or suspicion about new providers, and/or struggle with disorders that may have high risk behaviors that impact the provider's safety (e.g., an individual with a neurocognitive disorder who is experiencing hallucinations and increased agitation).

Let Others Know Where You Go

Depending on your connection to a team, it is always prudent to let others know where you are going or devise a strategy to allow others to access your travel schedule. In the case of Veterans Affairs, some government vehicles are outfitted with tracking technology that allows the hospital site to track where the car is and how long it has been in a specific location. In cases of concern, it may be possible to collaborate with your garage team to ask for additional oversight and monitoring of your car's whereabouts, and length of stay. For those not connected to an organization, providers can create confidential travel logs that detail their travel plans, or use phone tracking technology to let others know their whereabouts.

Develop and Socialize Your Policies

It is wise to have thought through what you will and won't tolerate regarding pets, weapons, and other behavior. Creating or identifying policies that align with safety goals is key to establishing safe practices. Policies should identify specific behaviors that are required by the patients in order to receive care (e.g., removing weapons from the therapy area, locking them up, and/or using safety locks), and specific outcomes should patients not comply with these policies (e.g., they do not receive care if they are in violation of the agreement). These discussions are not punitive, but rather can be integrated into part of the informed consent process and/or a behavioral plan or treatment contract. In cases where there may be some concern prior to going to the home, these requests can be discussed over the phone.

Identify Your Own Internal Compass

Dr. Hendrik was consulted to see a male patient who was 57 years old and unmarried and lived with his brother. He was referred by his nurse, who indicated that the patient had uncontrolled diabetes, and only indicated that he had a "strange" relationship with his brother. The referring nurse had a history of providing unsafe referrals, was known to cross boundaries with patients, and tolerated violations of company policy (e.g., open weapons in the home). The patient lived in a remote area, in a rundown home, with poor cell-phone service.

Upon carefully entering the darkened home, Dr. Hendrik noted several open boxes of cereal on the table, and used diabetic syringes strewn haphazardly across the kitchen counter. She could see a figure lurking behind a boarded wall, supposedly the patient's brother, and notably a large pit bull was chained to the couch with a rusted chain-link leash. The dog appeared friendly, but was straining at the leash, while the patient slapped at his back and yelled at the dog to lay down on the couch.

After introductions, Dr. Hendrik continued to note a personal sense of unease related to her safety, something she had not felt in her three years of providing care in the home. The referral question was not clear, the environment was not entirely transparent. Knowing her unease was masked by her professional demeanor, it continued to grow as the patient interrupted the assessment several times to reassure her that she was safe, and that he was not going to hurt her.

It is important to identify written policies, but it is also important to review one's own personal limits with safety. Sometimes, there will be situations that raise the hair on the back of your neck. It is acceptable and appropriate to act on one's instincts, and usually unease is driven by something more concrete than what is identified in the moment. In the scenario above, it is perfectly acceptable for Dr. Hendrik to trust her instincts and leave the home, not to return. Exploring trends in her reactions may allow her to understand any biases she may have, but Dr. Hendrik also had the experience to know that something did not seem right. In the cases where the provider frequently struggles to tolerate even occasional safety challenges, struggles to set clear and firm boundaries, or is not ready to accommodate the extra work of managing home safety concerns, they may not be best suited to this type of work.

If working for an organization, it can be uncomfortable to assert one's need for personal safety and adhere to policy. Sometimes, organizations have external pressure or demands that do not align with policy or personal comfort. For example, there may be specific census requirements that result in more lenient practices by supervisory staff who aim to increase productivity or revenue. The culture of a work team, or a supervisor who does not understand home care, may also have a negative impact on the referral process and put social pressure on the MH provider to comply with violations of policy, cross boundaries, or disregard safety measures. Being self-aware, and aware of your company policies, and finding support from like-minded colleagues, can help you identify your own internal compass and conduct yourself in a safe manner. Ultimately, you will need to advocate for yourself and your team, and this a fundamental aspect of practicing safely in home care.

Being Aware (Once You Are There)

For all MH providers, part of the job is to be aware and observe one's surroundings. In home care, this observation begins as you approach the home. Taking in your surroundings and being aware of the environment are essential to detecting and addressing any concerns that may arise. Consider any environmental obstacles or dangers (e.g., exposed wires, holes in the ceiling, black mold, ice or snow) and observe the state of the home you are entering.

It is not necessary to have your first conversation with the patient inside the house. If you have specific concerns, it is acceptable to identify yourself prior to entering the home and have a preliminary conversation with a patient on his or her porch or entryway. This conversation will allow you time to examine environmental concerns as well as specific patient concerns. As the MH provider, you can assess the presentation of the patient, affect, and level of agitation and orientation. You can determine whether there are others present in the home, and the relation of those individuals. This will help you respond appropriately, prior to serious concerns arising.

Occasionally, you will stumble upon a crisis. A patient has fallen, and you are the first one to arrive; a patient is found unresponsive; there is drug paraphernalia, or weapons, lying about; a dog looks like it is about to attack you. These situations are relatively commonplace given the complex nature of geriatric home-based care. Here are some specific tips and tricks to managing these obstacles that arise.

Specific Tips and Tricks

Car/Transportation Safety

Your transportation is only as good as the vehicle in which you ride. It is important to make sure your vehicle is maintained, just like you would with a personal vehicle. If you have the luxury of a company car, you may be able to advocate for four-wheel-drive or snow tires. If you are using your own vehicle, it may be useful to invest in something that can meet your driving needs. Having a sense of how one's car handles challenges like ice, mud, or wind can help to make an informed decision on where you should be driving. Providers may want to have a basic working knowledge of their car, how to change a tire, and how to check oil, or identify someone they can call in case of an emergency. It is wise to ask one's company for a car safety kit, or purchase one if one is not available. In case of a breakdown or delay, having additional supplies, including food, water, and blankets, can be insurance against difficulty. For the sake of good customer service, it can be useful to find a confidential way to transport patient phone numbers (i.e., a locked briefcase) or have a way to contact administrative staff who can assist with letting patients know you will be delayed in the case of a vehicle breakdown.

Weather

Depending on your location, the climate can be quite variable. Being aware of your surroundings and whether you live in hurricane territory or are at risk of apocalyptic snow storms, and understanding the typical seasonal expectations of your environment is essential to preparation. There are several steps you can take to prepare for the weather:

• Check the weather forecast *before* you leave, especially if you are traveling long distances.
• Check the forecast of all the cities you will drive through, given that weather can change rapidly and vary from location to location.
• Dress appropriately. You may not always have access to air conditioning or heat, so taking care to dress in a way that will not put you at risk of overheating or being too cold is essential. You may have to trudge through mud, gravel, or snow, so wear appropriate footwear.
• Always bring appropriate supplies, such as water, mittens, and ice-scrapers.
• Consider bringing a credit card or cash (especially if you are in a rural area and may not be able to use a credit card) for cases where you get stranded and may need money to stay overnight or get assistance.

Safety Considerations for Urban Environments

Providers working in urban areas must consider management of traffic and other aspects unique to more populated areas. If you work within a team, it can be useful to consult with others prior to the visit and request information about their knowledge of areas of the city. They may have important details about where to park, their experiences with neighbors, and any problems they may have encountered on the visit. If you do not have access to a team, you can familiarize yourself with multiple ways to enter or exit the street for the home you are seeking.

Some patients may not have a designated parking spot in their home or apartment complex. It is prudent to park your car in a well-lit and open area. While many cities may have strict parking ordinances, it is important to resist the temptation of parking in an alleyway or in tight parking spots between buildings that local residents suggest using. When this happens, the provider may end up being blocked in by delivery trucks or other vehicles, making it difficult to leave or increasing the risk of an accident. Sometimes vehicles with special markings, such as a government license plate, may draw the curiosity and attention of neighbors and other residents. It is often best to keep a generally low profile and only disclose your identity to those who need to know.

There are several factors to consider when visiting large apartment complexes and senior housing facilities. Make sure to carry appropriate identification. Many facilities have intercom systems to allow visitors access to the building, while others may have attendants or security at the front desk who may require you to sign in. It is recommended that you contact patients via telephone a few minutes prior to your arrival to inform them that you will be using the intercom system. Use professional judgement when riding in elevators with other residents in the building. While it might cost you a few minutes from getting to a visit on time, it is an investment in your personal safety and patient confidentiality. You may want to take a moment to familiarize yourself how to access alternative entrances/exits.

Managing Pets

Being comfortable with animals and pets is a helpful but not necessary part of home care. Generally, most pets are domestic animals that are friendly around humans, which is partly why they are considered pets. This is not always the case. The provider will want to determine whether there are pets in the home, in part because it may be disruptive to the therapeutic process, but also to determine whether there are any safety concerns. Here are some general ideas about how to manage pets:

- Find out if the patient and/or family has a pet, and remind them to secure pets prior to your visit.
- Consider integrating a policy about pets into part of your informed consent and therapy agreement.
- Once you arrive, if the patient forgot to secure the animal in a different room, ask the patient to do so prior to entering the house.

Of course, having a certain comfort level with animals is helpful, as providers will be exposed to a great many pets of different types and breeds. Depending on your assessment of the situation, you ultimately may have to adapt. Providers have been known to allow friendly pets to sit on their laps during therapy sessions rather than repeatedly remove them during the session. Some providers may even bring treats or toys, but this may encourage boundary crossing, de-emphasize the professional nature of the visit, and increase any risk and liability (i.e., what if the animal does not tolerate the treat or toy?). Thus, we recommend avoiding these practices.

Weapons

Depending on the cultural environment of the area where one works, there may be varying attitudes towards and/or reasons for weapons to be in the home. In more rural areas, it may not be surprising to have a confused patient greet a provider with a hunting rifle or have a small gun on the coffee table for shooting squirrels, or to notice a large collection of guns above the patient's mantle. In some cases, weapons may have a symbolic meaning the patient may want to discuss with a provider.

As previously mentioned, it is important to be aware of and socialize company policies and laws related to management of weapons in the home. Neurocognitive difficulties can increase the risk of injury to those that have access, and it is recommended that clinicians regularly screen for access to firearms (Betz et al., 2018). The provider can assess by phone whether the patient has weapons in the home prior to arrival, and remind the patient to put weapons away before meeting. Upon arrival, it is acceptable to ask the patient to put away weapons if they forgot. Agencies like Veterans Affairs may supply gunlocks, and these can be provided to patients at no cost. For patients that have advancing dementia, it may be best to speak with a family member about safe storage strategies. Finally, enforcing policies related to weapons, and making patients aware of what those are, are key to maintaining safety.

Medical Safety

Most agencies require a basic level of life-support and/or first aid training. Having a basic level of awareness of how to respond in a crisis situation can be helpful in saving a patient's life. Below is a list of actions to consider for medical safety:

- Get basic training (CPR, first aid) and keep appropriate medical supplies in your vehicle.
- Be aware of resources in the area (fire or police departments).
- Be aware of whether you are in a no-cell service area, and know where the patient's landline is in the home.
- Consider being trained to use naloxone (Narcan), and have a way to access it, especially for patients with opioid prescriptions.
- Know patients' emergency contacts prior to arrival.
- Have phone numbers of the patient's medical provider (if possible).
- Understand infection control protocols for patients with contagious illness by talking with medical staff.

Substance Use/Abuse

While behavioral issues related to substance use and addiction do occur in outpatient clinic settings, working with patients in their home that are under the influence of alcohol or narcotics can present its own set of challenges. Many home-based programs have policies about providing care to patients that are intoxicated. In many cases, providing medical care may run counter to therapeutic goals of treatment, alter vital signs, or interfere with lab results. Therefore, education about substance use treatment is warranted, and it is important to assess whether the patient's personal safety is at risk.

While clinicians have varying amounts of experience and training in substance use disorders and addiction, it is important to understand how treating these issues in the home is quite different than an inpatient setting. Providers are vulnerable due to the lack of additional staff support, and the patient's potential access to weapons, and are sometimes in locations far from emergency services. Not all patients that have substance use problems exhibit violent or other inappropriate behavior. Consider the following options when providing care to patients that have been identified as having a substance use issue:

- Consult with other disciplines who have recently seen the patient, and inquire if the patient was under the influence of drugs or alcohol during the visit.
- Call the patient just prior to the visit to determine if there are signs of impairment due to substance use, including slurred speech, agitation, or euphoria.
- Inform another staff member or program director of your visit with the patient and consider having this person contact you at a designated time.

- Define the limits of your willingness to enter a patient's home if they are intoxicated.
- Conduct visits with teammates and assess the patient for safety and eligibility for or interest in services.
- Reschedule the visit if you arrive for a visit and they are intoxicated.

Home Oxygen

Dr. Hendrik arrived at Mr. Aquino's rundown apartment in a small city. Mr. Aquino was a 65-year-old man who had bipolar disorder with psychotic features, as well as diabetes, coronary artery disease, and chronic obstructive pulmonary disease. He smoked three packs of cigarettes per day and was oxygen-dependent. Mr. Aquino was friendly but suspicious, often set off by providers he felt were not listening to him. After a productive therapy session, Mr. Aquino followed Dr. Hendrik out to the porch of the apartment complex, his oxygen in tow, chatting about his upcoming medical appointment. With his oxygen still on and nasal cannula in place, Mr. Aquino smoothly pulled out a cigarette and lit it.

Tobacco smoking has been identified as one of the greatest risks for individuals who use oxygen (Cooper, 2015). National data indicate that 83 percent of injuries from burns related to use of home-oxygen therapy were due to smoking (Assimacopoulous et al., 2016). Individuals sustaining burns from home-oxygen therapy are often older (M = 63.9 years) and are at greater risk of respiratory failure, mechanical ventilation, and pneumonia compared to non-home-oxygen therapy burns. Data examining the prevalence across four states of fatal fires associated with smoking indicated that the overall fatality rate was 3.8 deaths per 10 million people (Centers for Disease Control and Prevention, Pelletier, & Wendling, 2008). Tobacco smoking and use of home oxygen is controversial, as it raises ethical concerns, and concerns related to withholding treatments from individuals suffering from an addiction. There are several preventative steps that can reduce the occurrence of injury or death from oxygen-related fires (Cooper, 2015):

- Help the patient with smoking cessation efforts.
- Ensure that the patient has appropriate safety devices added to their oxygen concentrators.
- Request a fire risk assessment for the home, by the provider responsible for the ordering or supplying the oxygen.

- Educate patients and caregivers on the risks related to home oxygen and fires.
- Establish policies that promote safety for the patient and those around them, consulting with a legal team.
- Encourage patients to have fire extinguishers and working smoke alarms.

Unwanted Physical Contact or Sexual Advances

Although unwanted sexual advances are never appropriate, for individuals with an incipient dementia inappropriate sexual behavior is common. Understanding the nature and context of the patient's behavior is important in determining one's response to it. Are you going to the home of a convicted sex offender? Or are you doing a neurocognitive evaluation of an individual with Alzheimer's disease who may be terminated from his day program because he tries to inappropriately touch his female nurses? Sometimes inappropriate sexual behavior is a result of a progressive neurocognitive disease; at other times, it is a well-established pattern of perpetration. The provider can find out some of this information prior to visiting the home. There may be public records, documented issues in the medical record, or even an involuntary termination of services from other agencies (like home health aides) due to inappropriate behavior.

Unlike other medical disciplines, the practice of mental health and the therapeutic relationship does not, and should not, involve touching. In fact, assessment and treatment can occur several feet away from the patient, which allows the provider to maintain physical distance that can be advantageous in working with a patient who may have a history of making sexual advances towards providers. In addition, the home environment lends itself to informality and familiarity. How you dress and behave can help promote the professional and therapeutic framework. Unwanted sexual advances can be stressful and traumatic, which is why it is important to take safety precautions. In cases where there is a known history, if you determine it is safe to go to the home there are several things to consider:

- State clear boundaries. You can let patients know that you will leave if you are threatened or if they are inappropriate.
- Go with a colleague, to curb the patient's behavior through social pressure and accountability.
- Choose where you sit wisely. You can sit near the door, or sit outside if possible.
- Involve partners or family members in treatment.

Managing Safety with Family Members or Other Members of the Community

Unlike working in a traditional clinical environment, clinicians in home-based care face the challenge of managing a variety of people that may or may not have any connection to clinical care. Family members, personal care assistants, neighbors, friends, and service providers may be present in a home during a visit at any time. This can make for challenging and awkward situations in which a provider is placed in the position of balancing the need for privacy and maintaining social graces that help sustain rapport. Being aware of any potential risk factors posed by others in the home due to mental illness, substance use, or a history of criminal behavior is an important part of forming strategies to cope with any potential problems with others in the home during visits. While these other individuals can be helpful at times to collect more information and understand our patients better, they may also have their own reasons for or intentions regarding interacting with providers. Consider these strategies when interacting with others in the patient's environment:

- Inquire about existing relationship dynamics within the patient's family, caregivers, and friends with other staff members prior to an initial visit.
- Limit discussion and interactions with other service providers in the home.
- Discuss the limits of being able to provide services in the home if there is a person present that is intoxicated, psychotic, or sexually inappropriate, with patients early in the therapeutic relationship.
- Apply the same principles of attending to personal safety as discussed earlier in the chapter with people in the home other than the patient.

Summary

In general, the incidence of difficulties in home care is relatively low. However, the risk associated with home care is higher than in an outpatient setting, due to the numerous obstacles that may arise. Anticipating the variety of challenges that arise on a typical day of home-based work is essential in managing those risks. Adequate preparation, understanding oneself and one's team, and being ready to react in case of an emergency are all key aspects of managing safety concerns on the road.

References

Assimacopoulous, E. M., Liao, J., Heard, J. P., Kluesner, K. M., Wilson, J., & Wibbenmeyer, L. A. (2016). The national incidence and resource utilization of burn injuries sustained while smoking on home oxygen therapy. *Journal of Burn Care and Research, 37*, 25–31.

Betz, M. E., McCourt, A. D., Vernick, J. S., Ranney, M. L., Maust, D. T., & Wintemute, G. J. (2018). Firearms and dementia: Clinical considerations. *Annals of Internal Medicine, 169*, 47–49. doi:10.7326/M18-0140.

Centers for Disease Control and Prevention, Pelletier, A., & Wendling, T. (2008). Fatal fires associated with smoking during long-term oxygen therapy–Maine, Massachusetts, New Hampshire, and Oklahoma, 2000–2007. *MMWR: Morbidity and Mortality Weekly Report, 57*(31), 852–854.

Cooper, B. G. (2015). Home oxygen and domestic fires. *Breathe (Sheffield, England), 11*(1), 4–12. doi:10.1183/20734735.000815.

7 Addressing Hoarding in Home Care

Michelle E. Mlinac

Mr. Sousa is a former chef who is meeting with his home care psychologist and social worker to talk about selling his home and moving to a smaller apartment. Dr. Olson and Ms. Leonard had met Mr. Sousa three months earlier for the first time and found him living in squalid conditions. He had been a caregiver for his parents, who had owned a restaurant where he had also worked. The home was filled with thousands of cookbooks, recipes, and kitchen appliances. The fire department has been to the home several times and the county health department was now threatening to condemn it. Mr. Sousa maintains two storage units full of items from his parents' and grandparents' homes that he wants to continue to maintain, though the monthly charges strain his already limited finances. In the three months since they met him, Dr. Olson and Ms. Leonard had helped him obtain heavy-chore services to begin a slow process of decluttering the home. Mr. Sousa is reluctant to move to another residence, but recognizes that he may not have much choice in the matter.

Late-life hoarding disorder (HD) is a challenging issue that can be driven and maintained by complex psychiatric, cognitive, and functional factors. These cases can become overwhelming to provider and patient alike. Safety of staff entering the home is critical, and precautionary measures should be taken to ensure care can feasibly be provided within the cluttered space. Animal hoarding may co-occur and can cause additional distress and health precautions for providers. In fact, patients with severe hoarding may never receive routine medical home care as they will likely opt out or avoid home visits altogether. However, they may end up involved with Adult Protective Services (APS) or undergoing guardianship proceedings and require capacity evaluations. Mental health providers in home care have a unique vantage point in being able to assess and provide treatment to those challenged by HD. This chapter provides a brief survey of assessment and intervention approaches to HD and offers suggestions for further resources.

Assessments

Clinical Interview

A clinical interview around hoarding behavior should explore the patient's perception of the problem, the onset, and precipitating factors, and, perhaps most importantly, identify the patient's own terminology used to describe the clutter. For example, some patients may want to use the term "stuff", others like "junk", and others may have their own preferred term. Aligning with a patient's terminology can be critical in building rapport in order to further address their hoarding behavior. Learning about the onset of hoarding may provide clues as to how the problem can be improved. For example, a different treatment plan may be required for a clutter problem that developed after the onset of cognitive or functional decline or after downsizing to a smaller apartment compared to someone who has been hoarding since childhood, and for whom HD runs in the family. Assessing for comorbid psychopathology is crucial, particularly for post-traumatic stress disorder, depression, obsessive compulsive disorder (OCD), substance use, and suicide risk. Life course and cohort factors can also impact treatment planning. For instance, patients who lived through the Great Depression or other situations of scarcity may have developed a pattern of loss aversion, hanging onto items "just in case" they are needed when resources are few. Hoarding behaviors may have the greatest impact on family, friends, and neighbors, and result in social isolation.

Functional Assessment

A functional assessment including activities of daily living/instrumental activities of daily living (ADL/IADLs) and the impact of clutter can be important for identifying other areas of concern. For example, an older adult may have the skills to cook for themselves, but if all meal preparation areas are covered with clutter, they may need assistance in obtaining adequate nourishment.

Home Safety Assessment

The provider should also assess the home environment, including fall risks or other hazards. A risk-assessment screen may include identification of areas where the clutter impedes exits, complicates medication adherence, or poses fire/electrical hazards. Counterintuitively, in homes with high amounts of clutter, patients may come to rely on certain areas to hold onto while walking to support them, and thus fall risk may still be present (or worsen) after clutter is removed. Safety issues should be addressed up-front to determine if care can safely be provided in the home. In extreme cases of self-neglect, the patient may need to be referred for emergent medical evaluation and/or to APS.

Hoarding-Specific Assessments

Brief hoarding assessments can be useful, and several are validated for older adults. The Clutter Image Rating Scale allows the examiner to understand how the patient sees the extent of the clutter in their home. The patient is shown a photo array of sample rooms (e.g., a kitchen) being gradually filled with clutter, and asked to identify which photo most closely matches the severity of their own clutter. Anecdotally, when using this tool during visits in hoarded homes, it is often quite startling to see the discrepancy between the patient's view of the hoarding severity and that of the provider's, while standing together in the midst of the clutter. This tool, which has been validated with older adults (Dozier & Ayers, 2015), can serve as a good starting point for treatment as providers can adjust their own understanding of the problem prior to embarking on an intervention pathway. The Savings Inventory-Revised, a 23-item self-report scale that aims to quantify intensity and frequency of hoarding behaviors, has also been shown to be valid with older adults who hoard (Ayers, Dozier, & Mayes, 2017).

Functional Analysis

It is critical to assess the person's process of accumulating items (and to understand if there are limited financial resources to do so). While some adults receiving home care are unable to bring new items into the home, others may be frequent shoppers at thrift stores, order items online, or collect items they encounter as they go about their days. Financial issues may be present, including unpaid bills, fees to maintain storage units, fines from landlords or the city, etc. Consider conducting a functional analysis of how items are brought into the home, how they are maintained in the home, and what barriers are present to removing items from the home.

Neurobehavioral Status Examination

A neurobehavioral status exam or neuropsychological assessment can help identify cognitive issues that may be perpetuating the clutter. Attentional impairments (including underlying learning or attentional disorders) and executive dysfunction in particular may interfere with the ability to sort and discard. Having an understanding of potential cognitive dysfunction may inform intervention strategies.

Independent Living Capacity Evaluation

Finally, independent living capacity evaluations may help determine a person's ability to remain living safely in the home or to make determinations about their future living situations. See Chapter 11 for more information on capacity evaluations in the home.

Interventions with the Patient

Psychoeducation

Psychoeducation may be the first line of intervention, and the International OCD Foundation (hoarding.iocdf.org) offers resources to teach the patient, family, and healthcare team about HD.

Motivational Interviewing

Next, engage the patient in motivational interviewing around readiness for change, specifically that "change" may be allowing a homemaker or heavy-chore service to begin coming to the home. Reframing the problem as the clutter being a barrier to healthcare may help to make it a smaller, more manageable problem that can be addressed step-by-step. For example, the provider and patient may choose to prioritize creating a safe path so that providers can enter the home, or work on clearing a space on a table so a nurse can fill a medication planner.

Psychotherapy

For older adults who can participate, formal psychotherapy is also an important tool. One approach for older adults developed by Ayers and colleagues (2014) paired exposure exercises with cognitive rehabilitation to address aversion to reducing clutter and challenges in planning and carrying out decluttering behavior. Cognitive behavioral therapy for depression and anxiety may be useful when indicated, and may be a good starting point for older adults who are reluctant at first to directly work on decluttering. Addressing underlying bereavement and trauma issues associated with the clutter may also be warranted, as in the earlier example with Mr. Sousa. Excellent treatment resources are available, including *Buried in Treasures* (Tolin, Frost, & Steketee, 2013), *Treatment for Hoarding Disorder: Therapist Guide* (Steketee & Frost, 2013).

Psychopharmacology

Psychopharmacological interventions, such as selective serotonin reuptake inhibitors, may reduce symptoms that exacerbate hoarding. Referring for a psychiatric evaluation can be useful. For patients who already receive psychotropic medication management in a clinical setting, it is important to ensure treating providers understand the severity of the hoarding problem.

Working with Family/Caregivers

Working with involved caregivers and family can be helpful, particularly around future planning or potential housing relocation. It can be prudent to identify any local support groups for those with HD, or their loved ones. Sometimes the clutter is not the patient's own but instead is from someone they live with, or is caused by both the patient and the family. In these cases, establishing workable and realistic goals together is key to avoiding staff burnout or worsening patient distress.

Working with the Healthcare Team

Within the context of a home care team, caring for a patient with HD can be challenging. Care provision in hoarded homes can be even more taxing, complicated, and risky than home care usually is. Offering in-service training to team members around HD may help to first provide basic education and dispel myths around HD. An interdisciplinary assessment (e.g. nursing, physical or occupational therapy, social work, mental health) can help inform the team's expectations and develop an inter-disciplinary treatment plan. A harm-reduction approach may help both patient and team to establish mutual goals of care; for example, reducing the risk of falls and improving medication management.

Consulting with Other Service Providers or Agencies

While there is little evidence that one-time clean-ups have any long-term efficacy for resolving HD, they may be necessary to address severe situations, particularly if the home is uninhabitable. Depending on where you practice, you may or may not have direct access to services to clean up within the home. If you are not able to offer such services, it is critical to partner with Area Agencies on Aging or other service providers who can offer services like heavy-chore or home-making that can provide more intense cleaning. Agencies may have access to grants or other funding meant to address hoarding issues, and can be leveraged to help the patient remain in-place safely. Consider informal mechanisms such as volunteers, church groups, or others in situations where time and resources are limited. Professional organizers can also be vital in helping the patient establish new routines for managing clutter in the home.

Landlords, apartment managers, and others who have ultimate ownership over hoarded spaces can be critical partners in clean-up efforts. Different states can offer a range of support. An example of best practice, masshousing.com has many resources that can assist those who are overseeing hoarded homes and apartments in the state of Massachusetts. Severe cases may also involve agencies such as APS, Departments of Public Health, or legal entities, in which your role may be to support and advocate for the patient, and to help guide interventions that are person-centered and empathic. In some jurisdictions, these agencies may be able to access funds or grants specifically earmarked to help those with HD.

References

Ayers, C. R., Dozier, M. E., & Mayes, T. L. (2017). Psychometric evaluation of the saving inventory-revised in older adults. *Clinical Gerontologist, 40*, 191–196.

Ayers, C. R., Saxena, S., Espejo, E., Twamley, E. W., Granholm, E., & Wetherell, J. L. (2014). Novel treatment for geriatric hoarding disorder: An open trial of cognitive rehabilitation paired with behavior therapy. *American Journal of Geriatric Psychiatry, 22*, 248–252.

Dozier, M. E., & Ayers, C. R. (2015). Validation of the clutter image rating in older adults with hoarding disorder. *International Psychogeriatrics, 27*, 769–776.

Steketee, G., & Frost, R. O. (2013). *Treatment for Hoarding Disorder: Therapist Guide (Treatments that Work)* (2nd ed.). New York: Oxford University Press.

Tolin, D., Frost, R. O., & Steketee, G. (2013). *Buried in Treasures: Help for Compulsive Hoarding* (2nd ed.). New York: Oxford University Press.

8 The Social Worker in Home Care

Donna Reulbach and Fred Pasche

Mr. Lang is a 94-year-old divorced man who lives alone in a dilapidated suburban house. The house is overgrown with shrubs and weeds and the front porch is overflowing with items that his daughter Jill has rescued from other people's discards. The yard and driveway are also piled high with old appliances and miscellaneous lawn ornaments and tools. The inside of the home is similarly filled to the brim with mail, magazines and books. Paint and wallpaper are peeling off the walls, windows are covered with old newspapers. The kitchen table has piles of mail 2 feet high and all surfaces are similarly overflowing with miscellaneous papers. Mr. Lang has managed to keep pathways clutter-free so he can get to the refrigerator and microwave and to his hospital bed in the dining room. Mr. Lang is in relatively good health but has severe arthritis which impedes his ability to walk safely and he hobbles along holding onto furniture or, occasionally, with a cane. The last time he left his home was one year ago because he fell and called 911. Mr. Lang was evaluated in the emergency room (ER). He had no injuries and was discharged back home. Mr. Lang has refused home health services but does accept help from a neighbor, Sandy, because he has known her for many years. Sandy does weekly grocery shopping and laundry, but Mr. Lang will not allow any other help.

Whose Life Is It Anyway?

At the core of social work practice are two fundamental principles: the right to self-determination and meeting a person "where they are." To adhere to these principles, social workers must manage challenges to boundaries, handle the complexities of family meetings, and coordinate with family and community partners. Respecting these principles can, as in the case of Mr. Lang, be both literally and figuratively challenging. It may be difficult for a provider to sit with Mr. Lang in his cluttered and unclean space, challenging to accept he has chosen to live in that environment. Given these challenges, human service professionals who chose to work with patients in a home-based setting may self-select into this work environment. It is prudent to examine one's own personal comfort with a scenario like Mr. Lang's.

Clinically, Mr. Lang's case is rich with opportunities to do interesting and satisfying work. Commonly conducted by social workers, a psychosocial assessment could include a rich mix of personal and mental health history, knowledge of what he enjoys and values, and current life stressors and coping skills. Armed with this information, the social worker can support Mr. Lang's choice to live the life *he* wants, while simultaneously helping him – through objective encouragement, flexibility, professional problem-solving skills, and empathy – to live the best version of that life possible.

An Ongoing Debate: Self-Determination

Mr. Roy is 97 and lives alone in a cluttered and neglected ranch home he built himself. He never married or had children and other than his home care team has no social support. He has one known relative, a cousin whom he has not spoken to in ten years. After a fall at home, Mr. Roy was hospitalized and discharged, with his consent, to a skilled nursing facility for short-term rehabilitation. Citing his poor living conditions at discharge, the rehab staff expressed concern about him returning home and questioned his independent living capacity. At the rehab, he was deemed to lack capacity for independent living and healthcare decisions, and his health care proxy, his cousin, was invoked and recommended placement in a long-term care (LTC) facility. Mr. Roy vehemently disputed the capacity decision and steadfastly refused LTC placement, strenuously advocating for his discharge back to his home. Mr. Roy's home care team, including the team psychologist, disagreed with activation of the proxy, and felt that he should return home under their care.

Given this context, the home care team along with the social worker became an advocate for Mr. Roy in asserting his wishes to his cousin. He had always been a fiercely independent person. The home care team felt strongly that if he were forced to remain in a nursing home he would be very unhappy and agitated. As a result, he would likely require constant behavioral management, eventually lapsing into an irreversible failure-to-thrive. The team also wanted to honor his long-held wish to remain at home. Though his home situation was not ideal, for Mr. Roy it represented the values of autonomy, independence and resilience that gave his life purpose and meaning.

Ultimately, Mr. Roy's cousin supported his return home. This case illustrates how difficult it can be to determine capacity when working with home-bound older adults. Each side was genuine in their belief that their judgment was correct. The debate between safety and self-determination is often an ongoing one, driven by the multiple constantly evolving factors that govern a person's physical and emotional well-being. The ethos of honoring and protecting an individual's right to self-determination is a primary tenet of social work practice, and social workers may be at odds with other health care professionals whose professional codes are more driven by the "do no harm" ethic. Providers who are drawn to home care practice may be more comfortable with a blurred line between safety and self-determination. In reality, some home-bound patients may live on that line indefinitely.

Boundaries

Ms. Brown is an 89-year-old widow who lives alone in her family home, where she has lived her entire life. Ms. Brown had meaningful yet strained relationships, including an emotionally intense marriage to her wife, who died three years prior. Ms. Brown is estranged from her two daughters, who are both in their late sixties, and who, given their mother's temperament, never found a sustaining emotional connection to her. Ms. Brown had felt supported by her wife's constant presence and attention. They were both artists who had intellectually rich and interesting lives they reveled in sharing with each other.

Since her wife's death, Ms. Brown has become extremely disruptive to the community. She constantly seeks help from anyone she can reach by phone, including the local police. In these regular calls she states she is in emotional distress or that she believes someone has taken personal belongings she later finds. This same help-seeking behavior has extended to her social worker, who identifies with Ms. Brown in a particularly personal way from her own history.

At 89, living alone with mild cognitive impairment, Ms. Brown is genuinely vulnerable, and her social worker assists with arranging for a full array of home services and adaptive equipment. Though Ms. Brown's practical needs are being met, she is still constantly calling her social worker, often at night and on the weekends, in emotional crisis. Joining with the team psychologist, who also sees Ms. Brown, the social worker has taught Ms. Brown emotional coping techniques. Still, these techniques do not always suffice. The setting of boundaries remains an ongoing task, as the social worker seeks to balance her own boundaries against her concern for and desire to help Ms. Brown.

For home care professionals, including social workers, the issue of boundaries can be challenging. What one professional may feel is an appropriate boundary, another may perceive as boundary-crossing. These are common judgements that must be made in home care. Social workers should be aware when involvement is beyond conventional boundaries, and be able to identify a reason why they are choosing to go that extra distance. If one cannot articulate a reason, or begins to lose sight of it, the social worker should re-evaluate his or her behavior. If not, patient care can begin to feel onerous, contributing to burnout and creating a dysfunctional rather than strong and helpful connection between social worker and patient.

Having a person in your professional environment whose judgement and counsel you trust is key to helping you maintain a healthy perspective and appropriate patient boundaries. This consultant, whether they be a colleague or supervisor, may notice (even when you don't) that boundary-crossing is becoming problematic.

Going with the Flow: Family Meetings

Mr. Pak, a 78-year-old, was facing a terminal medical diagnosis. He had a history of alcohol abuse but continued to have the support of his eldest son. Mr. Pak was not thriving at home, though he retained decision-making capacity, and had previously expressed his wish to stay, and die, at home. Given his complex medical issues, his quality of life at home was poor. A family meeting was held with Mr. Pak, his son and the home care team. Both he and his son were nodding during the meeting, but said very little, despite the many questions being posed to them.

In family meetings, social workers often have varied and shifting roles, including the role of a mediator, assisting with setting limits, being a surrogate listener, modeling healthy communication and protecting patients and families. In Mr. Pak's case, because he and his son had little experience with complex medical situations, they were unaware of important follow-up and clarification questions. They also may have felt too intimidated or awkward to ask them. In this instance, the social worker played the role of surrogate listener and questioner, modeling ways to interact with the medical team. The social worker helped ensure that Mr. Pak and his son understood the medical information by asking the team questions on their behalf, saying, "I'd like to make sure I'm understanding this," which allowed the patient to have his needs met while saving face and not being put on the spot. Because of this intervention, Mr. Pak was then able to articulate what quality of life meant for him in that moment. His son then worked with the team to support his father's end-of-life goals.

Coordination with Providers and Community Partners

As social workers, our work often involves collaboration and cooperation with providers in the community; with home-bound clients this collaboration is essential. Many of our patients need assistance from a variety of resources, such as Elder Services, food stamps, housing, rehabilitation centers, inpatient hospitalizations, mental health services and other community agencies. Developing a relationship with local Elder Service agencies is vital, as they are often the key player as the provider of elder services for a cluster of communities. They are knowledgeable about other community services and often have a myriad of programs designed to help older adults age in place.

It is also important to follow patients as they transition from home to hospital to rehabilitation; meeting in person may not always be feasible, but contact with the team social worker in various settings often elucidates aspects of the patient's life that are not apparent in the inpatient setting.

> Mr. Greene is a legally blind, 78-year-old, man who lives alone in an assisted living facility (ALF). He receives daily meals at the facility and has a home health aide who assists him five days a week. Mr. Greene has mental health conditions that have been stable for many years due to an effective mental health treatment team. Suddenly, Mr. Greene refused the assistance of his aide with his showering. The next day he appeared disheveled and confused, so the aide consulted with the ALF staff and Mr. Greene was sent

to the ER. The home care social worker reached out to the ER social worker and later to the inpatient social worker to provide history and describe the patient's baseline in the community. The inpatient team was considering placement in an LTC facility. However, the home care social worker was able to describe the patient's living situation as a supported, stable and safe environment. This critical collaboration among social workers allowed the patient to avoid placement and return home with close follow-up by the home care team.

Consulting Adult Protective Services

As mentioned earlier, self-determination allows our patients to make their own choices, some of which may expose them to risk or danger. When does the right to make unhealthy choices cross the line to self-neglect or even abuse? The patient will often deny the need for intervention because they value their independence or because they rely on the help of the abusive caregiver and are fearful of losing this connection. When considering if a situation reaches the level of requiring an Adult Protective Services (APS) report, a social worker should consider the following:

- Does the patient have the capacity to make her/his own decisions?
- Is the patient aware of the risk or danger that they are exposed to?
- Is the patient willing to accept services to ameliorate the conditions?
- Does the situation pose an immediate, serious threat to the patient's safety?
- What are the local mandates and laws about reporting?
- What might happen if a report is not filed?
- What is the assessment/perspective of other members of the interdisciplinary team or other providers?

If safety concerns warrant the filing of an APS report, social workers are mandated to report regardless of the wishes of the patient. Throughout the relationship with the patient, concerns about the patient's safety should have been discussed with them in a way they could understand. Similarly, if an APS report is being filed, the social worker should explain to the patient (and if appropriate, the family) the action being taken and the protective service process, so they know what to expect. The home care social worker ideally can "team" with the APS social worker to develop a plan to keep the patient safe in the home.

In this chapter, we have described the responsibilities of a social worker as case manager with an aging, home-bound population. However, social workers often provide other services in the home. For end-of-life care, hospice services are provided by an interdisciplinary team including social workers who also offer bereavement counseling for the family after the death of the patient. Social workers can also provide advance care planning or advance directive discussions. In the case of a court-appointed guardian, social workers often partner with attorneys to offer case management and therapeutic counseling to the person receiving guardianship services. The role of the home-based social worker is multi-faceted and rewarding. At the same time, it can be a challenging balancing act negotiating ethical issues and maintaining healthy therapeutic boundaries. A supportive system of colleagues and maintaining connections to professional organizations (www.socialworkers.org, www.swhpn. org) can be helpful.

9 The Psychiatric Provider in Home Care

Marc Nespoli

As a geriatric psychiatrist you have been asked to make a home visit to see Mr. Young, who is 84 years old and lives alone. Mr. Young's wife died six months ago, and though he still drives there is concern about his safety in doing this. He has also lost weight, and his hygiene has been poor, prompting concern about depression or dementia. On your visit, Mr. Young states he is doing "fine" since his wife died, he denies feeling depressed or anxious, and he has no thoughts of suicide or not wanting to live. His sleep is adequate, he stays active around the house during the day, and although he cannot explain his weight loss he says his appetite is good. Cognitive testing via the Saint Louis University Mental Status Examination is noted for a 20/30. Mr. Young reports being independent with his activities of daily living and instrumental activities of daily living (ADLs and IADLs). You note his house to be mostly clean, minus the bathroom, which is very unkempt. There is limited food in the refrigerator, but Mr. Young notes that he prefers to eat out for most meals. His car shows no signs of accidents, and his bills, while somewhat scattered, appear to be paid on time. Mr. Young has a history of not believing in taking medication, and so defends his medication non-adherence as a "personal choice." The only collateral contact for Mr. Young is a nearby brother, who states, "He is who he is, he has always done things his way and I'm not too concerned about him."

Although unusual for general adult psychiatrists, the above is a typical case for a geriatric psychiatrist who is able to make home visits. I have had the pleasure of serving in this role for a Veterans Affairs home-based primary care (VA HBPC) program over the past seven years. As I often tell the residents and fellows who rotate on our service, a geriatric psychiatrist making home visits has *in vivo* data available to them that cannot be realized in a clinic setting. Functional determinations are not based on the word of patients or family members—they are seen first-hand and, as this case demonstrates, are invaluable to the patient assessment.

The goal of this chapter is two-fold: first, I would like to provide a sense of the role of a geriatric psychiatrist who makes home visits. The experiences described are based on care provided in the VA, and a limitation of this chapter is the lack of comment on Medicare or private insurers. Second, I will describe typical clinical situations one might encounter with geriatric home visits. Although there are similarities to outpatient treatment, psychiatric house calls do have unique aspects which differ from the typical clinic visit.

Role of the Geriatric Psychiatrist in Home Care

As a geriatric psychiatrist, one must be very clear in defining the role within the home care team. Because psychiatrists in most states are differentiated from psychologists by having the authority to prescribe medication, your treatment relationship in home visits will be established, and guided, by this differentiation. In addition, within VA HBPC, the mental health provider role is more often filled by psychologists rather than psychiatrists; policies regarding evaluations and termination of care are often designed with this in mind. As psychiatrists, once a medication has been prescribed, we may not be able to admit and discharge patients from the home care program as efficiently as our non-prescribing colleagues.

The primary question to ask your home care team is whether you serve as a one-time consultant to the team, or a long-term treating provider for each patient you see. In our geographic catchment area, the average daily census for our home-based team is approximately 450 patients, which along with high patient turnover and driving distance can make evaluating and following up with every patient a difficult task. However, if one were to serve only as a consultant to the team, one could more easily perform one-time evaluations, or time-limited treatment. By not initiating prescription medications, one could then triage patients to the clinic or other community providers for further follow-up. I have chosen to adopt a hybrid model in which I will only see patients who have an active psychiatric issue or concern, and who are truly homebound due to physical, cognitive, or social reasons. I also make certain that patients will be on the program long-term, so I will not have to unexpectedly discharge them at some point in the future. It is important to understand this distinction, as it will influence both how you are utilized by your team and how you will manage your (ever-growing) caseload going forward.

To illustrate, I was asked to see an 80-year-old male patient with a recent stroke who was depressed and having passive suicidal ideation. The nurse seeing him on our home care team was planning to keep him long-term in the program, but because he eventually needed more services for his ADLs, he was discharged from our VA team to a Medicare visiting nurse association (VNA) (our local policy is that patients cannot concurrently receive both). I had started this patient on an antidepressant and a sleep medication, and because he was homebound I was not able to transfer him to the clinic or a community provider. Whereas I often relied on the VA HBPC nurse visiting him to update me on his status at weekly team meetings, I no longer had this reliable collaboration once the VNA took over. This naturally led to me needing to make more frequent home visits, taking time away from other patients. It is easy to see how this scenario could unfold for several patients concurrently, and lead to an accumulation of patients for psychiatric management who are no longer part of the original treatment team. Although there are times when these circumstances cannot be avoided, it is necessary for the psychiatrist to try and foresee all possible outcomes before committing to care for a patient in the home.

Psychiatrists in home care must also clarify if they will be acting solely as a prescriber, or also as a therapist. For those psychiatrists who have the benefit of a psychologist on their home care team, this is obviously not a concern. Unfortunately, our team does not have this luxury, and so although I enjoy being able to engage in therapy as well as psychopharmacology, I have learned to recognize the potential for this to create a role which might not align with your expertise.

For example, I was once asked to arrange a family meeting for a patient who reported his family to be "nagging him" about moving to an assisted living facility. Because I knew the patient possibly lacked capacity, I arranged for a family meeting so that I could gain collateral information from his very involved children. What I did not foresee, however, was that the family had a long history of in-fighting, and his placement was becoming another issue for the five children to disagree about. The meeting turned contentious, and from then on I was called continually by each of the children in order to hear their side of the story, and further put the patient in the middle of a difficult decision. In hindsight, I think this family meeting was probably better led by a social worker or psychologist. Their expertise in managing family dynamics and group therapy, as well as knowing more about the resources available to this patient, would have better served the family than mine. As a psychiatrist, if your home care team has psychologists and/or social workers who are able to engage in individual or family type therapy, it would likely be to your benefit to defer these types of visits to them.

The above are all examples of defining your role as a psychiatrist on a home-visit team. Because psychiatrists are often prescribers, they can be bound to patients in ways that other team members might not be, which can affect the team dynamic you are a part of. Also, and as has happened for me, you will find that once outpatient primary care providers and specialists learn of a psychiatrist who makes house calls, the referrals will come flooding in. This, too, will have implications for what criteria you might utilize in determining which patients are best served by psychiatric home visits.

Special Considerations for the Geriatric Psychiatrist Making Home Visits

Substance Abuse

Patients with substance abuse issues have been a challenging issue for our home-based program for several years. As psychiatrists we often manage substance abuse in the clinic, just as we do depression, dementia, or schizophrenia. Patients might be more likely to be under the influence of a substance when we see them in their home environment. This has led to staff safety concerns amongst our team members, and questions of whether there should be a policy of discharging those who are actively abusing substances. If there is such a policy, what defines active substance use—hours prior to visit? Days prior to visit? During the visit? Related to this, what if the psychiatrist decides to treat a home care patient who is substance dependent with naltrexone or acamprosate, and then your home care team discharges this patient from the program? As mentioned previously, you are still bound to that patient by prescribing for them, and so you could conceivably be required to continue to see them without team support.

High-Risk Patients

Similarly, patients who are considered "high risk" can be a cause for concern for the home care team, and especially the treating psychiatrist. In the clinic, we usually have the benefit of a nearby emergency room (ER), and the ability to coordinate a higher level of care for patients who are in crisis. With home visits, these options do not exist, at least not on-site. Instead, you need to call 911 or the police if you are visiting an acutely high-risk patient. Moreover, for patients who may not need an ER visit but do need a greater frequency of home visits, this is a challenge for a busy provider to accommodate. In the clinic it is easier to fit patients into 20- to 30-minute daily or weekly appointments as needed. For home visits, you may be driving long distances to a patient's home, which can make it difficult to meet the appropriate level of care for high-risk patients.

This challenge of having high-risk patients carries over to the team as well, and it may be your responsibility to decide who should and who should not be admitted to your program. For example, consider a homebound patient with major depression, borderline personality traits, and a long history of suicide ideation and attempts. Whereas I feel mostly comfortable with his risk assessment and management, it is naturally challenging for our nurses, physical therapists, and dieticians to manage the complex psychiatric needs for this type of patient. While the team may be less conservative with whom they treat, you must also consider the overall comfort and safety of the team on home visits when determining who is appropriate for the program.

Serious Mental Illness

Issues facing patients with severe mental illness (SMI) overlap with those of high-risk patients. Whether it be suicidal ideation related to depression, or florid psychosis from schizophrenia, patients with SMI often require a unique set of tools for their treatment plan. Many patients in this population need medication injections, multiple lab draws to check medication levels, EKGs to rule out antipsychotic QTc prolongation, or even electroconvulsive therapy. Although not impossible, many home-visit patients do not have easy access to these treatment modalities, and so one must consider this when deciding if the home setting is a safe and appropriate treatment venue for them, or if they would be better served in more traditional outpatient care.

Capacity Evaluations

Being asked to assess a patient's capacity to live at home independently is perhaps the most common request of a home-based geriatric psychiatrist. Although this question arises in the clinic as well, patients tend to be referred for home care because they are struggling to care for themselves independently, or there are issues involving home safety. Focusing on practical problem-solving solutions, which involve both the patient and team, should be the preferred plan of care in these situations.

For many years, our team had followed a 75-year-old man with mild cognitive impairment. His hemoglobin a1c was rising due to poor dietary choices and medication non-adherence, and he would often use the ER for routine, non-urgent needs. The outpatient primary care provider had become frustrated with these issues and wanted the patient to be found to lack capacity so that he could be placed in a nursing home, and at less risk for an adverse event. However, this patient valued his independence immensely and did not want to leave his home. Instead of making a "capacity determination," our team sat down with him, discussed the concerns, implemented a medication reminder system, and had him agree to a home health aide. All were instrumental in addressing the provider's concerns, and improving the patient's health and satisfaction. Although this is one of the simpler capacity evaluations, it illustrates how home care might push and pull you in different directions than you might normally have in a clinic setting. This is when it is helpful to rely upon the interdisciplinary team and use the home visit as a way to develop practical solutions which reflect the uniqueness of each patient. See Chapter 11 for further discussion of home-based capacity evaluations.

Summary

The above is a brief summary of the role of the psychiatrist, and situations commonly seen as a psychiatrist making home visits. Work in a geriatric psychiatry clinic can be like private practice, whereas work in the home setting is more akin to being in the Intensive Care Unit. The former will have you seeing many (mostly stable) patients throughout a typical day, while the latter will consist of fewer patients with greater clinical needs and acuity who require a whole team of providers to keep them well. The advantages to the latter setting are numerous—by seeing patients in their home environment, you get a wealth of clinical information, and you can put them at ease. This will lead to richer sessions, in a setting that differs from the monotonous pace and scenery of a clinic. Your patients and their family members will treat you as a welcome guest in their home, knowing you are committed to helping them safely age in place.

Part 3

Assessment and Treatment Considerations

10 Assessment Screening Tools and Approaches

Courtney O. Ghormley and James "Chip" Long

Mr. Buddy Joe Smith is a 78-year-old white male with a high school education who describes decreased motivation and increasing memory problems that have started to impact his daily activities. He has a history of cerebrovascular disease and Parkinson's disease, which have limited his ability to ambulate without a rolling walker. His medical issues have progressed to the point that he requires in-home assistance from both his spouse and home health aides.

Geropsychology is one of the most dynamic areas of psychology, largely due to the complex nature of the patient population it serves. As can be seen by the case example, patients referred to home care often have various comorbid diagnoses that impact their functioning on several levels. These types of complicated referrals are the norm, rather than the exception. As such, part of the role of the mental health (MH) provider in home care is to assist the treatment team in clarifying the interactions between the medical, cognitive, and psychiatric spheres. Data collected during psychological and brief neurocognitive assessments can play a vital role in piecing together the puzzle. Therefore, this chapter will focus on several techniques and processes that may be helpful while condensing the information gathered through clinical observations, formal testing data, and working with the patient's support system.

Purpose of Home-Based Testing with a Geriatric Population

Cognitive screening or a brief neurocognitive assessment provides information on the patient's cognitive abilities. Reports from the patient or family members regarding cognitive problems are helpful, but to truly assess a patient's ability there is no substitute for standardized measures. While the driving force behind testing is often diagnostic in nature, there are many other benefits to assessment. Assessment can be a valuable method of communicating the patient's cognitive strengths and weaknesses to team members and the family. Providing hard data on the patient's cognitive impairments can often help family members make the connection between the underlying cognitive limitations and the behaviors they observe. When this understanding is lacking, we will often hear such things from family members as "He knows what he is doing," "He could do it, he is just ornery," or "She has always been this way, and she really has you fooled." Testing provides an opportunity to explain the processes involved and provide education on the complexities of major neurocognitive disorders (MNCDs) to those involved in the patient's care.

The completion of a formal assessment can also help to clarify inconsistencies in the patient's clinical history. Often, we receive referrals for patients who have never been diagnosed with MNCD, but who have clear cognitive deficits during even the most surface conversations. The opposite is also not uncommon, where we admit a patient who has a current diagnosis of MNCD, but who performs well on brief mental status screening measures and remains involved in the management of instrumental activities of daily living (IADLs) (e.g. money management, medication management). While the MH field understands the importance of using psychometric data to make the diagnosis of MNCD, there can be a lack of understanding of the specific criteria in the larger health field. In some cases, we have seen a diagnosis of dementia placed by a primary care provider simply due to the patient's age and a self-report of memory changes. MH providers working with older adults should be aware of personal and professional biases such as this that may lead to misinterpretation of symptoms or a misdiagnosis due to a lack of critical clinical information.

Finally, a cognitive assessment provides necessary information for comprehensive treatment planning within the interdisciplinary team setting. The MH provider plays a notable role in the development of the treatment plan, both in the identification of goals and determining the most effective ways to meet these goals. One example might be recognizing the importance of medication adherence in managing the patient's health issues. While this seems elementary, if there are cognitive problems that could interfere with the patient's ability to meet this treatment goal then the MH provider can inform the team of this issue and assist in identifying compensatory strategies. Some options might include the following: utilizing an alarmed pill organizer, educating the family about the patient's memory limitations and the need for supervision, or leaving a written list of the patient's medications in the home so it can be referred to if there is a question. In order to fully maximize the treatment-planning process, the MH provider must be comfortable working with other disciplines. And while this is true for all MH providers in medical settings, it is especially true in the field of geriatrics. Understanding the interplay between medical and psychological variables when working with older adults is vital. MH providers can maximize this dynamic in such a way that optimizes the efficiency of the care provided to the older adult.

Practical Considerations for Conducting Assessments in the Home

Neurocognitive testing in the home has several unique aspects that differentiate it from a traditional assessment completed in an office setting. While efforts are made to remain true to the basics of the test administration, alterations in the process by which this is executed are common and often necessary given the setting. Additional considerations involve how to manage family involvement, compensate for hearing/vision deficits, and incorporate the non-psychometric data into the conceptualization process.

Non-traditional Sources of Information

As mentioned above, the information gathered from psychometric tests provides concrete data about the patient's abilities across multiple cognitive domains. An additional benefit of home assessment is the invaluable access one has to the peripheral information that can provide depth to the testing data. We have often joked that in our previous office-based jobs working with older adults, we were blissfully unaware of the need for the unfiltered information that comes from viewing how someone functions in their home.

Assessment begins when you call the patient to set up the testing appointment. Being mindful of whether they can track the conversation, whether their responses are congruent to the questions being asked, and whether they are able to remember the date and time of the appointment are all initial clues about their functioning. On the day of the appointment, we often call the patient before leaving the office to make sure they remember our conversation and are still available. This practice is based on our experience of having shown up to the home for a scheduled appointment, only to find the patient has forgotten it and made other arrangements (at the grocery store, at the doctor's office, etc.).

Additional information about the patient's cognitive and functional status is available when you pull up to the residence. Observing the condition of the exterior of their domicile can provide valuable information, even before you make it to the door. Oftentimes, due to the patient's declining health status, they are no longer able to maintain a home or yard in a way to which they are accustomed. This can result in feelings of depression and worthlessness, and often drives the most common concern we hear – "I just can't do the things I was once able to do." Being aware of these variables and making sure to incorporate them into the assessment is important.

Scheduling Considerations

Consideration should also be given to whether the clinical interview and neurocognitive testing should be completed in one session or broken up into multiple appointments. There are pros and cons for each approach, and we have taken both routes in the past depending on the circumstances. If the testing is completed in separate sessions, this allows for a more detailed intake assessment and minimizes patient fatigue. More time can be spent on an informal assessment of the patient's cognitive abilities and assessing the patient's accuracy when providing personal information from their history (previous occupations, prior dates of significant medical events, what was discussed when the nurse was last in the home). We have both noticed a tendency for our patients to spend a significant amount of time during the day watching TV news. Asking the patient questions about a specific current event can provide information on the patient's awareness and understanding.

Logistical Issues in the Home Testing Environment

One of the main challenges in home-based assessment is to locate a clean and quiet area for testing. Realize that the home setting is going to present unique challenges and be able to problem-solve in order to establish the best environment possible. Situations may involve helping the patient clear off the kitchen table for testing, and asking that pets be put in a different room. Balance assertiveness with respect and aim to put things back in place so you "leave it how you found it." Remember that you are a guest in the home.

Finding a suitable testing location also depends on the patient's functional abilities. Can they sit upright for the testing session? Are they more comfortable in their recliner? If they are bed-bound, is it a hospital bed that can be adjusted so that the head is raised and they can view the test booklet, or write? In this way, the provider must flexibly work with the patient to find a comfortable setup that also enables them to complete the necessary tasks.

There are many similarities between completing a bedside exam in a hospital and completing testing in the home. In both cases, the setup is likely going to be less than ideal and will necessitate adjustments in order to accommodate the patient's needs. We have each tested under unique circumstances – sitting on a patient's bedside commode because there was no other seating option and examining on the front porch of a home because the air conditioner was broken. In each of these circumstances, standardized test procedures were stretched to accommodate the situation. While not ideal, there are many times where these modifications are unavoidable. As a result, the clinician must have a flexible mindset in order to gather the most accurate data possible, while at the same time staying as consistent as possible to standardizations. If adjustments were made during the process of testing, these should be noted in the report, along with an opinion on whether they impacted the results in a clinically meaningful way.

Consideration of Sensory Deficits

When conducting an assessment within the home, the testing environment is often not optimal, and it will rarely be as conducive as that found in the clinic. The appointment should ideally be scheduled at a time when you are least likely to be disturbed (e.g. before young grandchildren come home from school). Depending on the home setting, there may be extra noise (i.e. a loud air-conditioning unit, street noise, a barking dog) or poor lighting that decreases the patient's ability to fully engage with testing. These factors are important to consider because the data gained from the assessment will be impacted by the amount of information (visual or auditory) that the patient is able to accurately perceive.

Vision and hearing impairment are common in older Americans. One in six people will experience visual impairment, and one in four has hearing loss (Dillon, Gu, Hoffman, & Ko, 2010). Sensory impairment is even greater among racial and ethnic minorities and among those living in poverty (Dillon et al., 2010). As such, it is important to assess this informally during testing. Prior to starting an assessment, it is important to inquire whether the patient wears glasses or hearing aids and if so, to encourage their use during the assessment. The patient's glasses may need to be first located and then wiped clean for the patient to see well. Lighting may need to be increased by opening the blinds or curtains or by bringing an extra lamp into the room. You may need to ask the patient's family or caregiver to turn off the TV or to turn down music in another room to create a quieter assessment environment.

If you note that the patient is having trouble hearing you or seeing the test materials, it may be helpful to use compensatory devices to optimize their sensory ability. If hearing is an issue, consider using a "pocket talker" or other amplification device. Often these devices consist of a portable microphone and headset that is worn by the patient to amplify sound (i.e. your voice) in the immediate area. If the patient is having difficulty seeing the test stimuli, consider the use of a magnification sheet. It can also be helpful to carry copies of larger-print stimulus pages for some testing measures. For example, the provider can easily increase the font of stimuli that need to be read by the patient or increase the size of photos used in naming measures.

If necessary, consider adjusting the assessment battery to compensate for the patient's visual or hearing limitations. This could include scaling down a larger battery such as the Repeatable Battery for the Assessment of Neuropsychological Status (RBANS) (Randolph, Tierney, Mohr, and Chase, 1998) so that items requiring vision are omitted for someone who has significant visual impairment. You can also consider using different tests developed for those with sensory impairment (i.e. MoCA-BLIND; Wittich, Phillips, Nasreddine, & Chertkow, 2010).

Managing Family Members

Not only does one need to manage various patient characteristics and the environment when conducting an assessment in the home, providers often must take into consideration the patient's family or caregivers. Spouses, children, grandchildren, home health aides, and others may be in the home when the provider attempts to conduct an assessment. It never fails that a random neighbor decides to drop by for a visit in the middle of the assessment. Managing these distractions during the assessment can have its own special challenges.

It is important to provide education about why the assessment is being completed to both the patient and the caregivers present. Unlike in the clinic, where we often whisk patients to a quiet room to be assessed while leaving their chatty family members in the waiting area, you may not have this luxury in the patient's home. It is important to ask the patient their preference as to whether they would like their family member to stay in the room. The caregiver may welcome a chance to relax or to attend to something else in the home, so it can help to give them explicit permission to leave during formal testing.

Often a family member will observe the assessment. This has its pros and cons. One positive aspect is that the family can observe that the patient is struggling with simple tasks (i.e. drawing a clock, making a block design). If a family member is struggling to accept that the patient may be experiencing cognitive difficulties, it may be helpful for them to observe it first-hand. Cons to consider when allowing family to observe the assessment include exposure to test content, alteration of the patient's performance, and risk of intrusion from the observer.

An important caveat: it never fails that a family member sitting in will attempt to cue the patient during the assessment. Often, they will offer prompts during a verbal fluency task, such as "Think about the animals in the zoo." They may shame the patient by saying, "Oh, come on! You remember that we went there on vacation 10 years ago!" Family members and caregivers do this for a variety of reasons. Notably, it is often difficult to see a loved one struggle with what should be a relatively simple task. They may want to protect the patient by offering support. There are also patients who will look to their family member in the room for help or assistance. You need to anticipate this and explain to observers that they must remain silent and that assistance cannot be given (no hints allowed!). It often helps to have the family member sit behind and out of the line of sight of the patient.

Information from Collateral Sources

Having a family member or caregiver provide collateral information about the patient's history and daily functioning can be extremely helpful. We often include the caregiver during portions of the clinical intake and later ask them about the accuracy of the responses provided by the patient. This provides a type of third-party review of the information provided by the patient. Sometimes this is best done after the session has been completed, to avoid embarrassing the patient if errors were made due to cognitive dysfunction. As mentioned above, there have been numerous times where the patient's caregiver has interrupted the process to confront the patient on inaccurate information provided to the clinician during the intake. While awkward, this provides an opportunity to describe how the patient's cognitive limitations can interfere with their ability to provide accurate information. It also gives valuable information on the depth of the caregiver's understanding of the situation, and how they approach the management of these issues in the home.

There are times when family members perceive that your assessment reveals significant deficits that are incongruent with the family's report about the patient's abilities. Why might caregivers overstate or understate the patient's ability? A spouse may report that the patient is still managing the finances and medications while your cognitive assessment reveals severe impairment in reasoning, memory, and executive functioning. This incongruence may relate to the caregiver's difficulty adjusting their own perception of the patient given the amount of time they have been with them. We have found spouses may "cover" for their significant other to hide cognitive limitations. This is often a surprise to other family members (i.e. children) when one spouse passes away and the remaining spouse struggles with tasks they are no longer cognitively able to manage. In other cases, the caregiver may offer a more impaired view of the patient's functioning than is evident from other sources. This may indicate that while the patient can rise to the occasion during testing, it does not reflect their typical behavior. It may also reflect caregiver burnout.

Types of Assessment

In home care, MH providers may be asked to provide a variety of assessments. The complexity of the assessment needed is often driven by the specific concerns or changes in functioning the patient is experiencing. In its most basic form, an assessment should include some sort of clinical interview to gather information about the patient's medical, psychiatric, educational, and social histories along with an understanding of their current functioning. Ideally a family member or caregiver will be present to provide collateral information. The clinical interview is often followed by administration of standardized measures of mood and/or cognition. The complexity of the assessment and the measures used can vary widely depending on the referral question and the training of the MH provider.

It is important to plan ahead, because you are limited to administering only the tests that you brought with you to the patient's home. For this reason, having standard psychodiagnostic batteries and cognitive assessment batteries is preferable. If there are unexpected results as you are moving through the assessment, then it might be necessary to make a return trip to the home. An alternative option is to keep a locked file in the trunk of the car with various testing instruments just in case another is needed at the time of the home visit.

Assessment of Mood and Anxiety

Mood and anxiety disorders are common among the geriatric population. The percentage of community-dwelling older Americans who have a mental illness, substance use disorder, or both, is roughly 1 in 5 according to a 2012 Institute of Medicine study (IOM, 2012). Blazer (2003) found that 1–5 percent of community-dwelling, older adults have major depression, and geriatric depression was associated with cognitive, social, and functional impairment. Anxiety is also common in older adults, with 7 percent meeting criteria for an anxiety disorder (Gum, King-Kallimanis, & Kohn, 2009). Notably, 27 percent of older adults seeking home care management experienced clinically significant anxiety (Richardson, Simning, He, & Conwell, 2011). Assessment of mood and anxiety symptoms often involves the use of standardized questionnaires to measure self-reported symptoms. When working with a geriatric population, it is important to select measures that have age-specific norms if possible (see Tables 10.1 and 10.2).

Assessment of Cognitive Functioning

MH providers are often called upon to determine if a patient has cognitive impairment. Brief cognitive screening measures require little time and can be used to provide a snapshot of global cognitive functioning. These measures are designed to be performed at the bedside if needed. While universal screening of cognition is not recommended, if a patient is experiencing signs or symptoms of cognitive impairment, cognitive screening can help determine the need for further assessment (see Table 10.3).

Brief Neurocognitive Testing

There are times when a more thorough cognitive assessment is necessary to provide valuable information about the patient's functioning or to

Table 10.1 Examples of Self-Report Measures to Assess Depression in Older Adults

Measure	Description	Considerations
Geriatric Depression Scale (GDS)	• Available in 15- or 30-item versions (Sheikh & Yesavage, 1986; Yesavage, Brink, & Rose, 1983)	• Dichotomous format (yes/no) • Easy to administer quickly with cognitively impaired patients • Heavily researched • Less somatic content
Beck Depression Inventory (BDI-II; Beck, Steer, & Brown, 1996)	• 21 multiple-choice, self-report items	• Strong psychometrics for geriatric population (Segal et al., 2008) • Challenging format for cognitively impaired
Patient Health Questionnaire (PHQ; Kroenke, Spitzer, & Williams, 2001)	• 2- and 9-item versions	• Validated with nursing home residents and geriatric community • Not extensively researched with diverse geriatric populations

Table 10.2 Examples of Self-Report Measures to Assess Anxiety in Older Adults

Measure	Description	Considerations
Geriatric Anxiety Inventory (GAI; Pachana et al., 2007)	• 20 self-report items • Agree/Disagree format	• Developed specifically for use with older adults
Geriatric Anxiety Scale (GAS; Segal, June, Payne, Coolidge, & Yochim, 2010)	• 10- (Mueller et al., 2015) and 30-item versions • 4-point Likert Scale	• Developed specifically for use with older adults • 30-item version provides Somatic, Cognitive, and Affective subscales
Beck Anxiety Index (BAI; Beck, Epstein, Brown, & Streer, 1988)	• 21 self-report items • 4-point Likert Scale	• Assesses common somatic and cognitive symptoms

Table 10.3 Examples of Cognitive Screening Measures Commonly Used with Older Adults

Measure	Description	Considerations
Montreal Cognitive Assessment (MoCA; Nasreddine et al., 2005)	• 30 items • Approximately 10 minutes to administer • Screens orientation, attention, executive function, constructional praxis, memory, language, and abstract reasoning	• Designed to detect mild cognitive impairment in older adults • Available in various languages • Version available for visually impaired
Saint Louis University Mental Status Examination (SLUMS; Tariq, Tumosa, Chibnall, Perry, & Morley, 2006)	• 30 items • Approximately 10 minutes to administer • Screens orientation, memory, mental calculations, attention, visual construction, language, and executive functioning	• Includes both list and contextual memory tests • Correlates well with comprehensive neuropsychological measures
Mini Mental State Exam (MMSE; Folstein, Folstein, & McHugh, 1975)	• 30 items • Approximately 10 minutes to administer • Screens orientation, memory, language, calculation, attention, and visual construction	• Widely used in the past, prior to the development of more comprehensive brief cognitive screening measures with better psychometric properties • Heavily weighted on orientation, which can fluctuate significantly in this population, especially in the presence of medical variabilities

Table 10.4 Examples of Brief Neurocognitive Tests Commonly Used with Older Adults

Measure	Description	Considerations
RBANS (Randolph et al., 1998)	• Approximately 30–45 minutes to administer • Alternate forms available • Assesses attention, language, visuospatial/construction, immediate memory, delayed memory	• Will need to consider supplementing with additional measure of executive functioning
Dementia Rating Scale – 2 (DRS-2; Jurica, Leitten, & Mattis, 2001)	• Approximately 15–30 minutes to administer • Alternate form available • Assesses attention, initiation/perseveration, construction, conceptualization, memory	• More appropriate for those with advanced levels of cognitive impairment

assist with making a diagnosis of a neurocognitive disorder. These types of assessment can be helpful in detecting dementia in patients. Brief neurocognitive testing generally provides an overview of the patient's performance on the following cognitive domains: Attention, Processing Speed, Language, Visuospatial Construction, Visual Perception, Memory, Executive Functioning, and Motor Functioning. A patient's performance on a screening measure may lead you to administer additional cognitive testing. For example, a patient may score well on a screening measure but still be reporting significant functional declines, or a patient may score much lower than expected on a screening measure but still be functionally independent. Your choice to pursue additional testing may be impacted by a variety of factors, including: the patient's prior level of education, English as a second language, the patient's mood or pain, or concern that the patient did not put forth enough effort. Brief neurocognitive tests provide a more in-depth look at the patient's functioning and can assist with diagnosis of MNCD and treatment planning (see Table 10.4).

In our home care practice, we are often called upon to assist with making a diagnosis of MNCD and to clarify a diagnosis. We often use a testing battery that includes a brief neurocognitive test supplemented by additional cognitive measures of language (i.e. verbal fluency), visuoconstruction (i.e. Block Design), executive functioning (i.e. Trails Making Test, Clock Drawing Test), motor testing (i.e. grip strength and fine motor skill), and mood assessments (i.e. depression and anxiety) to obtain a comprehensive picture of the patient's cognitive functioning.

Notably, not all MH providers in the home setting have been trained in or are comfortable with this level of assessment. In this case, referring the patient to a neuropsychologist for additional testing is highly recommended. Additionally, if you complete a brief neurocognitive assessment and feel that additional assessment is needed for clarification of diagnosis, referral for neuropsychological testing may also be warranted.

Summary

Completing an assessment in the home can be a challenge, for many of the reasons identified above. However, the clinical advantages of providing testing services in this setting far outweigh any difficulties you may encounter. We are hopeful that this chapter has outlined the value that psychodiagnostic and neurocognitive assessment can add to patient-focused geriatric home care.

Thinking back to the case example of Mr. Smith, completing a brief neurocognitive assessment could have yielded the following:

1   Provide Mr. Smith and his family with a better understanding of his overall abilities.

2   Clarify what type of compensatory strategies might help to maximize his functional status in the home.
3   Provide the medical team with information that could help determine the appropriateness of treatment recommendations (e.g. sliding-scale insulin) or equipment for the home (e.g. electric wheelchair).
4   Improve the patient and family's understanding of how the cognitive symptoms impact the patient's day-to-day functioning.

Any one of these benefits would justify the need for testing, and when you think more systemically about the data, the importance of this type of clinical assessment becomes clear.

Perhaps the most important benefit to this type of assessment is the opportunity to maximize the care provided to a patient population that is often overlooked or marginalized. In our experience working in geriatric medical settings, there can be a tendency among professionals to discount the importance of neurocognitive assessments in the sick or medically frail older adult. Often, this is rooted in the mistaken assumption that the testing "won't tell us anything we don't already know" or "won't change our approach to managing the patient's illness." Part of our role on the interdisciplinary medical team is to be an advocate for the patient's MH needs. Sometimes that involves providing education to the team on the clinical benefits associated with this type of testing. There is a need for each of us to continue developing skills in this area, as it is a vital part of providing comprehensive medical care to a geriatric population.

References

Beck, A. T., Epstein, N., Brown, G., & Streer, R. A. (1988). An inventory for measuring clinical anxiety: Psychometric properties. *Journal of Consulting and Clinical Psychology, 56*, 893–897.

Beck, A. T., Steer, R. A., & Brown, G. K. (1996). *Manual for the beck depression inventory* (2nd ed.). San Antonio, TX: The Psychological Corporation.

Blazer, D. G. (2003). Depression in late life: Review and commentary. *Journal of Gerontology: MEDICAL SCIENCES, 58A*, 249–265.

Dillon, C. F., Gu, Q., Hoffman, H., & Ko, C. W. (2010). Vision, hearing, balance, and sensory impairment in Americans aged 70 years and over: United States, 1999–2006. *NCHS Data Brief, 31*, 1–8.

Folstein, M. F., Folstein, S. E., & McHugh, P. R. (1975). Mini mental state: A practical method for grading the cognitive state of patients for the clinician. *Journal of Gerontology: Series B: Psychological Sciences & Social Sciences, 12*, 189–198.

Gum, A. M., King-Kallimanis, B., & Kohn, R. (2009). Prevalence of mood, anxiety, and substance-abuse disorders for older Americans in the National Comorbidity Survey-replication. *The American Journal of Geriatric Psychiatry, 17*, 769–781.

IOM (Institute of Medicine). 2012. The Mental Health and Substance Use Work-force for Older Adults: In Whose Hands? Washington, DC: National Academies Press.

Jurica, P. J., Leitten, C. L., & Mattis, S. (2001). *Dementia ratings scale-2: Professional manual.* Lutz, FL: Psychological Assessment Resources.

Kroenke, K., Spitzer, R. L., & Williams, J. B. (2001). The PHQ-9: Validation of a brief depression severity measure. *Journal of General Internal Medicine, 16*, 606–613.

Mueller, A., Segal, D., Gavett, B., Marty, M., Yochim, B., June, A., & Coolidge, F. (2015). Geriatric Anxiety Scale: Item response theory analysis, differential item functioning, and creation of a ten-item short form (GAS-10). *International Psychogeriatrics, 27*(7), 1099–1111.

Nasreddine, Z. S., Phillips, N. A., Bedirian, V., Charbonneau, S., Whitehead, V., & Collin, I. (2005). The Montreal Cognitive Assessment, MoCA: A brief screening tool for mild cognitive impairment. *Journal of the American Geriatric Society, 53*, 695–699.

Pachana, N. A., Byrne, G. J., Siddle, H., Koloski, N., Harley, E., & Arnold, E. (2007). Development and validation of the Geriatric Anxiety Inventory. *International Psychogeriatrics, 19*(1), 103–114.

Randolph, C., Tierney, M. C., Mohr, E., & Chase, T. N. (1998). The Repeatable Battery for the Assessment of Neuropsychological Status (RBANS): Preliminary clinical validity. *Journal of Clinical and Experimental Neuropsychology, 20*, 310–319.

Richardson, T. M., Simning, A., He, H., & Conwell, Y. (2011). Anxiety and its correlates among older adults accessing aging services. *International Journal of Geriatric Psychiatry, 26*, 31–38.

Segal, D. L., Coolidge, F. L., Cahill, B. S., & O'Riley, A. A. (2008). Psychometric Properties of the Beck Depression Inventory—II (BDI-II) Among Community-Dwelling Older Adults. *Behavior Modification, 32*(1), 3–20. https://doi.org/10.1177/0145445507303833.

Segal, D. L., June, A., Payne, M., Coolidge, F. L., & Yochim, B. (2010). Development and initial validation of a self-report assessment tool for anxiety among older adults: The Geriatric Anxiety Scale. *Journal of Anxiety Disorders, 24*(7), 709–714.

Sheikh, J. I., & Yesavage, J. A. (1986). Geriatric Depression Scale (GDS): Recent evidence and development of a shorter version. *Clinical Gerontologist: The Journal of Aging and Mental Health, 5*(1–2), 165–173.

Tariq, S. H., Tumosa, N., Chibnall, J. T., Perry, M. H., & Morley, J. E. (2006). Comparison of the Saint Louis University mental status examination and the mini-mental state examination for detecting dementia and mild neurocognitive disorder – A pilot study. *The American Journal of Geriatric Psychiatry, 14*, 900–910.

Wittich, W., Phillips, N., Nasreddine, Z. S., & Chertkow, H. (2010). Sensitivity and specificity of the Montreal Cognitive Assessment modified for individuals who are visually impaired. *Journal of Visual Impairment and Blindness, 104*, 360–368.

Yesavage, J. A., Brink, T. L., & Rose, T. L. (1983). Development and validation of a geriatric depression scale: A preliminary report. *Journal of Psychiatric Residents, 17*, 37–49.

11 Capacity Evaluations in the Home

Michelle E. Mlinac and Jenny Yen

"I'm too tired to see you today. I want to rest." Mr. Martinez had said these exact words the day before when he declined to allow me in for our testing appointment. Only this time, he believed he was saying it for the first time.

Once again, I stood before Mr. Martinez in the same poorly lit hallway lined with mundane, homogeneous forest-green doors. This time, I did not offer to accommodate him by coming back again tomorrow. Instead I stated, "This [testing] bag is so heavy, would you offer me a seat to sit down?" It appeared as if a lightbulb went on in Mr. Martinez's mind. He swung open the door and gestured for me to sit on a metal chair next to a commode.

I walked into his modest 8 ft by 10 ft home, a single-resident occupancy, and did a 360-degree scan of the room. At this moment, my priority was not to assess his home environment, but to get to know him as a person. There were no personal photographs or ornaments of any kind. However, his white walls displayed magazine cutouts of notable African American figures such as Tyra Banks, Michelle Obama, and Oprah Winfrey. I took my time and admired each art piece while he watched me. I shared my observations with him about how well cut out the photos were and how the women wore colorful attire. He smiled, and he shared his appreciation for beautiful, strong women. I also expressed my appreciation for how his artful display evoked a vibrancy in his home. He nodded respectfully toward me. We began forming a relationship from his beautiful displays of prominent African American women.

When I sat down, I took several mental notes on how he was living and functioning based on his home environment. The room was relatively organized and uncluttered, though everything looked stained and worn down. His bed was covered with loaves of bread and jars of peanut butter and jelly. He shared about his love for PB&J sandwiches ever since he was a little boy. I noted a couple of scattered frozen TV dinners labeled "fish" that were no longer frozen. Mr. Martinez sat down on his battered-looking twin-size bed that had stained, crushed cardboard boxes laid atop it. I realized that he was using cardboard boxes as incontinence pads, despite having several new packaged pads stacked in a corner.

There was a small sink and a metal shelf below a tiny mirror. The shelf was lined with a toothbrush, Pepto-Bismol, and Tylenol. There were no prescribed medications or a pillbox in sight. However, there was an unopened, over-the-counter ointment for toothache and gum pain relief near his bedside. I asked Mr. Martinez if I could examine this medication, to which he agreed. He shared that someone, though he could not remember who, had dropped it off. I asked if he had any tooth or gum pain. He smiled and used a dirt-stained finger to touch the back of his mouth. He said, "It only hurts if I touch it." He proceeded to touch it five more times. Although he winced every time, he would laugh softly and expose the few teeth he had remaining. This was the beginning of my evaluation of his capacity to make medical decisions.

Unique Aspects of In-home Capacity Evaluation

When we have asked older adults served in home care about their goals, they often say their main priority is to "stay home" rather than being moved to a new environment (e.g., a skilled nursing facility or their children's home). That aim may come into conflict with the often very valid concerns by others in their lives that the home is becoming an unsuitable place for them to live. This dilemma may raise questions of the person's capacity to remain in their home, make decisions about their care, or manage their financial resources. Conducting capacity evaluations with medically complex older adults who may have limited resources can be challenging. The outcome of these evaluations can have very serious implications on a person's legal rights and future. Ethically, mental health (MH) providers must balance the person's right to self-determination against risks to their well-being. Clinical judgments of capacity should be data-driven and prioritize the person's safety and well-being, while personal biases are best kept to a minimum. Providing these types of evaluations in the person's own home offers the MH provider the opportunity to conduct a more holistic and naturalistic assessment than might be possible in a hospital or clinic setting. In order to foster person-centered outcomes, we often start these types of evaluations by asking the question, "What does 'home' mean to you?"

This chapter examines the complex issues in home-based capacity evaluations. The purpose of this chapter is not to recreate capacity assessment guides that are described more thoroughly elsewhere (e.g., American Bar Association and American Psychological Association Assessment of Capacity in Older Adults Project Working Group, 2008), but rather to explore issues that are particular to this complex patient population and milieu of assessment. We will describe two of the ways that MH providers can conduct these types of evaluations, within a team context or as an independent contractor. Of note, for consistency's sake we use the term "patient" to refer to the individual who is being given the capacity evaluation. In some cases, depending on the role of the MH provider and the auspices in which testing is occurring, this person may not actually be the MH provider's patient, and this should be clearly explained prior to the evaluation.

Complexity of the Population

By virtue of having care delivered in the home, patients may be more complex than those typically seen in an outpatient setting. These patients are often medically ill with multiple chronic conditions and functional limitations, including treated or untreated cognitive impairment, that make it burdensome for them to access medical services in outpatient clinics. Although in-home services help to increase access to healthcare for this vulnerable population, the MH provider faces unique challenges when testing in an unpredictable environment. Patients served in the home may have limited stamina for long testing batteries or are frequently hospitalized, making it tricky to schedule home visits when they are medically unstable.

When working with severely impaired patients who may not have seen a primary care provider for several years, the MH provider's task can be even more challenging. These patients likely have undiagnosed or untreated cognitive impairment, MH issues, and chronic and acute medical conditions. Patients may be so impaired that they cannot function safely in their homes, manage their activities of daily living/independent activities of daily living (ADL/IADLs), or maintain a sanitary living environment, which may result in self-neglect or financial abuse. For example, patients may be living in a rodent- or bug-infested home, having their water or electricity shut off, being served eviction notices, or be a victim of a financial scam.

Addressing Referral Questions

A common referral for a capacity evaluation is a request to assess a person's "competency", which is a legal rather than clinical determination, and a frequently misused term. This generalized referral often requires the MH provider to follow up with the referring party for further clarification and education. Referring parties are often unfamiliar with appropriate terminology (*competency* vs. *capacity*) or use *capacity* as a catch-all word. Although this offers a wonderful opportunity to educate the referring party, the MH provider must also dig deeper by inquiring about a patient's presentation and circumstances, and discerning what type of capacity evaluation the referring party may actually be looking for. Referrers may not have an understanding of the full scope of the situation, and more risks may not reveal themselves until the MH provider visits the home to begin the evaluation. For example, the MH provider may observe the patient eating spoiled food or notice the accumulation of unopened mail.

In our experience, the most common capacity evaluations conducted in the home setting are medical decision-making, financial decision-making, and capacity for independent living. A person's capacity for medical decision-making may be questioned when they have repeated emergency room visits and hospitalizations, poor management of chronic or acute medical conditions, or poor adherence to medication management. A person's capacity for financial decision-making may be questioned when they have forgotten or refused to make a payment (e.g., rent, utility, file taxes). A person may also have difficulty writing or mailing a check, or have mismanaged their funds or been susceptible to financial abuse or scams. Questions about capacity for independent living may arise when the home setting is hazardous, or when a person's needs no longer fit with the environment in which they are living.

Due to the frequent physical, cognitive, MH, and functional complexities inherent in this patient population, multiple capacities may be requested to be evaluated at the same time. For example, the referring party may request a medical decision-making capacity evaluation, but upon entering the home the MH provider may note obvious home safety hazards or witness the patient responding to telephone scams. In some cases, it may make sense for the MH provider to adjust their approach and address multiple capacities at once. In other cases, the parameters of the MH provider's job may be to focus on the original capacity in question and then follow up on other issues at a later date. Capacity can fluctuate, and often may need to be re-evaluated over time.

Obtaining Records

Medical record reviews are a crucial portion of a thorough capacity evaluation. Reviewing records is a crucial aspect of the evaluation that helps to orient the assessment, compare findings from previous assessments or from a patient's baseline functioning, review medication regimens that might affect cognition, and rule out any underlying medical or MH issues that may be contributing to their presentation (American Bar Association and American Psychological Association Assessment of Capacity in Older Adults Project Working Group, 2008). The trajectory of the patient's history is crucial to understanding their current context. In settings like the VA (Veterans Affairs) where a long medical history is commonly stored in an electronic health record, the challenge can be to pick out information germane to the capacity report from among what can be lengthy notes from many providers.

In other settings, patients may not have robust medical records to review, or their histories may not be readily accessible. Due to MH or cognitive issues, or limited access to or a general distrust of healthcare systems, patients may not consent to release their medical records or may decline to disclose personal information, or they may have limited medical information to review due to inconsistent care or being lost to follow-up.

When compared to an MH provider who works for an institution, a major barrier for an independent contractor in completing assessments is obtaining medical records. In these instances, an independent MH provider could request that the referring party provide *any* information they have on the patient. It may be time-consuming, but there may be relevant information when sifting through the referring party's documentation. It is also important to state any limits in available records in the written report to demonstrate sound practice and professional competency. Furthermore, having limited access to records makes for another strong advantage in conducting in-home evaluations where there is an increased reliance on the patient's current functioning and behavioral observation in a patient's home environment.

Efficient Rapport-Building

In contrast to testing in a hospital or clinic, the power dynamic between patient and provider is shifted in the home and ultimately the provider is a guest there. A major barrier for the MH provider providing in-home capacity evaluations is being invited into the home, particularly when a person with advanced cognitive impairment does not remember the MH provider nor the purpose of the visit. The ability to form and convey a genuinely caring relationship on the spot is essential to overcoming this barrier. As in the case of Mr. Martinez, the MH provider was intentionally mindful in getting to know him over the course of the evaluation as opposed to solely focusing on the assessment process. By doing so, the MH provider demonstrated genuine care and built a trusting relationship by exploring his interests, appreciated how he personalized his home, connected with him around his valuing strong women, and integrated humor with the patient's long-time fondness for PB&J sandwiches.

Similar to other successful psychological interventions, assessments, or treatments, a strong rapport with one's patient is the heart of that success. A strong rapport may be developed based on Rogerian principles of a person-centered approach in which the MH provider must demonstrate active listening, empathetic understanding, and unconditional positive regard toward the patient. This creates a caring relationship fueled by openness, trust, and collaboration, which allows the MH provider to be welcomed in the home even when the patient does not recall the MH provider nor the purpose of the appointment.

A key way to quickly build a trusting relationship is to use positive, nonverbal language, such as a friendly smile and open arm gestures (as opposed to crossing one's arms, holding a clipboard, or keeping one's hands in one's pockets). Taking some quality time getting to know the patient's interests or actively listening to a favorite anecdote prior to testing helps to convey genuine care for the patient's well-being, values, and personhood. If the patient is familiar with the referring party or another provider on their healthcare team, this can also be helpful to share with the patient, as it provides important context for obtaining informed consent.

Consent vs. Assent

While a strong rapport is a catalyst for a patient to experience recognition and validation, it also helps in putting a patient at ease toward testing, and encouraging them to make their best effort and sit through lengthy batteries that are often uninteresting and mentally exhausting. It may also elicit buy-in from the patient to consent or assent to participation in the capacity evaluation. While informed consent "requires that one's consent to treatment be competent, voluntary, and informed" (ABA & APA, 2008, p. 19), a patient with untreated, advanced cognitive impairment may not have the cognitive ability to consent to participation in a capacity evaluation. Providers are highly encouraged to provide informed consent by explaining the rationale, purpose, benefits, and risks of a capacity evaluation in simplistic language to obtain assent. However, providers should not feel discouraged or falsely take on owner- ship of having to assess a patient's capacity even if a patient does not consent or assent to the capacity evaluation. It is important for providers to respect a patient's autonomy to decline testing. Referral sources should also understand that providers who provide in-home testing are not the only party responsible for making decisions regarding a patient's capacity, though home-based assessments are an attractive option to support patients in a least-restrictive environment. There are a couple of alter- native options if a patient does not consent or assent to testing. The MH provider may offer a clinical opinion about a patient's capacity without their participation in testing by compiling evidence based on observation in the home, behavioral observations, record review, and/or collateral interviews. Another option is that a patient is involuntarily hospitalized, and capacity may then be evaluated by a qualified professional in that setting. Thus, there are multiple avenues to meet the care needs of this complex population. In-home healthcare is just one way to provide care with dignity, and to preserve a patient's independence for as long as possible and in a non-institutionalized setting.

Home Setting

When compared to the traditional clinic setting, home-based testing affords several advantages and additional complexities. First, patients being examined may be more comfortable and at ease in their own homes, supporting a more optimal performance. Having patients demonstrate their best performance is important for all assessments, but particularly critical when a finding of lacking capacity may result in a patient losing certain rights and liberties. Clinic performance may not readily translate into what actually happens at home. Ecological validity can be enhanced by directly observing patients engaging in the ADL/IADL tasks in question rather than using a proxy of simulated tasks that might be done in a traditional clinic setting. For example, a semi-structured functional test in the clinic may be used to approximate how a patient might mail a letter, dial 911, or remember to take medications, but directly observing a patient performing these tasks in their everyday environment is much more valuable, and is ultimately what providers are trying to evaluate. Alternately, barriers that are apparent while observing the patient do these tasks in the home may not be present in a controlled clinic setting. For example, a patient may be able to sit with a clinic pharmacist and be coached fairly easily into being able to pack a medication planner, but have problems when translated into the home setting, where old pill bottles and medication planners may distract and complicate the task.

There is also an opportunity to gather information relevant to the capacity finding that may not arise from a traditional clinical interview. A next-door neighbor may stop by to bring lunch to the patient and share that they keep an eye on the patient and provide other needed supports. These types of informal social relationships may not fall into the role of formal caregiving (and thus may not be identified as such in an interview), but the patient may actually have a network of informal helpers that play a role in supporting the patient in ability to live independently.

Completing financial capacity evaluations in the home can also be advantageous over a clinic-based exam. For example, it is not uncommon to find evidence that a person has become a victim of a financial scam through mail or similar paperwork. Older adults may receive an alarming amount of daily mail, including solicitations for both real and fraudulent charities, sweepstakes, or other appeals for money. Alternatively, the MH provider may observe the deft skill with which the patient thwarts a telemarketer who calls during the exam. Similarly, a patient who is difficult to reach to schedule appointments, or never seems to listen to voicemails or return messages from providers, may actually be trying to avoid telemarketers rather than being non-adherent with care. In these cases, the MH provider has the opportunity to witness and probe further about the patient's understanding and judgment regarding such scams.

In contrast, there are drawbacks in conducting capacity evaluations in the home. Chaos often reigns, and inevitably the phone will ring during the free-recall portion of a memory exam. Psychological tests are not typically normed for use in the home; thus, this should be considered during interpretation. In addition, general logistical challenges are frequently encountered, such as not having a table on which to complete a paper-and-pencil task or place testing stimuli.

Given the amount of information one can get through observation, taking time to survey the environment can be very beneficial when ultimately making these challenging and complex determinations. An informal observational survey of the home may note these general themes:

- Hazards (clutter and fall risks, non-working smoke and carbon monoxide detectors, accessible access to rooms and exits).
- Communication (working landline or cell phone, internet connectivity, how well they are managing their postal mail and bills).
- Self-management (food, laundry, medications, and who is managing this if not the patient).
- Personal effects (photos, hobbies, care they have put into their space, and why it is important).
- Immediate outside environment (security, neighborhood, stairs, elevator, access).

One of the biggest hurdles may be having limited time to perform the capacity evaluation. The MH provider is encouraged to carefully consider which test to administer first because there may not be enough time to utilize all the tests that one had initially planned. We recommend maintaining a flexible approach, being prepared if necessary to change the order of tests administered. The goal is to obtain as much crucial information as possible, without overburdening the patient with tests that are not germane to the referral question or that have been answered by other information evident in the home environment. Capacity evaluations can be stressful and fatiguing for the patient being examined, so exams should be prioritized to be focused and precise.

Report Findings and Recommendations

Conducting capacity evaluations in the home allows providers to have a well-rounded picture of the patient's immediate circumstances, and thus to communicate these observations to others who do not have this vantage point. While providers are not generally providing an exhaustive list of in-home observations, it is important to capture relevant aspects of the patient's surroundings and distill these findings into meaningful information for those reading the report. As with many evaluations, it is important to ground recommendations in the patient's strengths and values.

Determination of capacity should be written clearly and explicitly, which in most cases will mean stating that in the provider's opinion, the patient either does or does not have capacity for the domain in question. If the provider's clinical opinion is that a patient has limited or diminished capacity, the provider is highly encouraged to specify in which type of situations would a patient have the capacity or not have the capacity to make a decision. For example, a patient may have diminished capacity for medical decision-making, in which he or she has the capacity to consent to simple medical treatment (e.g., getting a flu shot), but does not have the capacity to consent to complex medical treatment (e.g., surgery). In another example, a patient may have diminished capacity for financial decision-making, in which he or she has the capacity to manage pocket money (e.g., twenty dollars or less), but does not have the capacity to manage larger bills or larger financial transactions (e.g., rent, utilities, check-writing, credit cards, or investments).

Recommendations can enhance the capacity conclusion, as well as the quality of life, treatment, and healthcare of the patient in the future. Providers should be creative and flexible in considering how the patient's values and performance on testing may be translated into real life. In our experience, sometimes solutions and opportunities that were not available at the time of the evaluation may emerge after the finding of incapacity. In cases of independent living capacity, healthcare providers may not be in a position to relocate the patient themselves. Instead, they may be working directly with an activated healthcare agent who has been empowered to make decisions on the patient's behalf. Therefore, recommendations in the report may include ways to support both the healthcare agent and the patient when dealing with these challenging circumstances.

In-home Capacity Evaluation: Two Examples

We next discuss two possible contexts for MH providers conducting in-home capacity evaluations, based on the unique settings in which the authors have worked.

Capacity Referral from within the Healthcare Team

The home care interdisciplinary team are meeting to review their care of Ms. Jackson, an 85-year-old African American former high school math teacher who had a stroke four years earlier that resulted in major neurocognitive disorder due to vascular disease. Her nurse provider says she is concerned that Ms. Jackson is failing in the home. The team's social worker concurs, saying he believes they have reached the limit of what in-home services are available to support Ms. Jackson to age-in-place. The physical therapist on the team is more optimistic and notes that Ms. Jackson has improved her mobility in recent weeks. The nurse has found Ms. Jackson more confused during the past two home visits and the dietician notes she has lost 10 lbs in a month. The team has not been able to identify any family or friends to provide additional support. The pharmacist reflects that the team have been caring for Ms. Jackson for three years and seem to be stuck in the same dilemmas about her care at every quarterly team meeting. They are wondering if it is time to formally assess her independent living capacity.

When the capacity question is being raised by an interdisciplinary care team in which the MH provider is a participating team member, the MH provider has the advantage of a more longitudinal view of the patient, and of the team's ability to provide care. This type of team (for example a home-based primary care or home hospice team) has often built a long-standing and collaborative relationship with a patient over time, and is well-positioned to inform the capacity evaluation with its own assessments and observations.

Interdisciplinary assessments can be highly beneficial as collateral data to inform capacity evaluations. Consider the following examples of input that can be obtained from the interprofessional team, and note this is not an exhaustive list:

- Nurse: ADL/IADL assessments, medication adherence, fall risk.
- Dietician: Dietary intake, diabetes self-management, nutritional self-neglect.
- Pharmacist: Ability to self-manage medications, medication review, minimizing side effects.
- Primary care provider: Complexity and understanding of medical information, response to goals of care discussion and other treatment decisions, medical problems that can impair functioning.

- Social worker: Available formal supports, appraisal of family/care-giver ability to provide support, need for input/referral to Adult Protective Services (APS), financial self-management and resources.
- Physical, occupational, and speech therapists: Overall functional ability in multiple domains, including home safety, self-care, and ability to learn new information, adhere to rehab goals, and adapt to functional changes.

Members of a well-functioning interdisciplinary home care team may be able to provide input on multiple types of capacity domains, and conduct their own empirical assessments that can support decisions of capacity retention or loss. Often these disciplines are evaluating patients on an ongoing basis, and these evaluations inform the overall patient care plan. The care plan is then adjusted to meet the needs of the patient, and the cycle continues over time (Feng, Murphy, & Mlinac, 2017). Individual team members, as well as the team overall, may have different levels of risk tolerance, which can also drive referrals for capacity evaluations.

In the home care team context, a good rule of thumb prior to pursuing testing is to encourage a team discussion about what will happen if the person lacks the capacity being evaluated. This can be particularly useful if the team are frequently requesting capacity evaluations for patients when it may be that the issue resides more with the team process or other issues like provider burnout. Due to the longitudinal relationship the team can develop with patients, team members may have strong feelings about the outcome of the capacity evaluation, regardless of what is determined. The MH provider's role may also include helping the team through their own feelings around determination of capacity or incapacity, and to determine what happens next in the context of what is in the patient's best interest.

In this longitudinal care context, the MH provider may also have the benefit of being able to offer support to patients, surrogate decision-makers, families, and the team following the evaluation. They can provide direct patient-centered feedback to these individuals and help to problem-solve issues that emerge after the capacity finding is made. They can work closely with the team's social worker to explore least-restrictive alternatives to enhance capacity or to assist with coordinating care with APS or other healthcare providers.

Capacity Referrals as an Independent Contractor

Through a partnership with an agency that serves older adults and dependent adults who have been reportedly abused, the MH provider may function as an independent contractor who conducts in-home capacity evaluations. This referral agency represents both the client and referral source. Through this transactional partnership, an independent MH provider's only role is to assess and offer a clinical opinion on a patient's capacity in the domain in question. When compared to an MH provider working within an interdisciplinary team, the independent MH provider cannot assess other areas of concern which may arise during the home visit. In addition, the independent MH provider would not make recommendations or interventions post-evaluation to further support the patient to stay in the home. There is no additional follow-up because guardianship or conservatorship is the last option at this point.

> Guardianship or conservatorship is defined as 'a relationship created by state law in which a court gives one person or entity (the guardian) the duty and power to make personal and/or property decisions for another (the incapacitated person) upon a court finding that an adult lacks capacity to make decision for him or herself'.
>
> (ABA and APA, 2008, p. 14)

Given the severity of this population, guardianship or conservatorship is likely the optimal pathway to support the patient's safety, general well-being, and quality of life.

Being an independent MH provider conducting capacity evaluations has several benefits and drawbacks. A major advantage in this role is being able to maintain a neutral and unbiased perspective when going into the evaluation; there is no external pressure from an individual or team for the evaluation to conclude one way or another. This unique role also offers exposure to a wide range of complex and intellectually stimulating capacity cases, as well as creative opportunities to refine one's assessment and rapport-building skills. Finally, the administrative aspects (e.g., billing, referrals) are outsourced to the partnered agency. A main disadvantage is the inherent challenge of a unidirectional partnership where communication is limited and there are few opportunities to improve the process. An independent MH provider also does not have institutional support or opportunities to consult with a team. A good rule of thumb is to stay connected with one's professional support system and continue networking by joining professional organizations or a consultation group.

References

American Bar Association and American Psychological Association Assessment of Capacity in Older Adults Project Working Group. (2008). *Assessment of older adults with diminished capacity: A handbook for psychologists.* Washington, DC: American Bar Association and American Psychological Association.

Feng, M. C., Murphy, M. R., & Mlinac, M. (2017). Independent living capacity evaluation in home-based primary care: Considerations and outcomes of quality improvement project. *Clinical Gerontologist, 40,* 51–62. doi:10.1080/07317115.2016.1210272.

12 Implementing Evidence-Based Psychotherapy in the Home

Julie Loebach Wetherell, Amanda R. W. Steiner, and Shannon Sisco

Evidence-Based Psychotherapy

In many ways, evidence-based psychotherapies (EBPs) are more appropriate and easier to conduct in the home than in other settings. The pressure to help older patients make important changes efficiently is greater when home care providers have fewer appointments per week than do outpatient mental health (MH) providers. Furthermore, therapy interventions can be tailored more appropriately when clinicians see the patient's environment, and a caregiver may be more readily available to enlist as a therapy coach. In this chapter, we describe how conducting EBPs in the home with older adults results in positive outcomes for the patient, the provider, and the team. We present case examples to demonstrate our work with patients as part of the Veterans Affairs (VA) home-based primary care (HBPC) program. In addition to describing empirically-based work for depression, anxiety, and insomnia, we also describe the process of including a caregiver as a therapy coach and using tele-mental health to conduct an EBP from a distance. Our primary goal is to demonstrate the benefits of providing EBPs in home-based care with older patients to in-home MH practitioners who typically use other therapy models.

"Evidence-based psychotherapy" refers to an intervention that has undergone scientific testing to establish its effectiveness. Usually this is done through randomized, controlled trials in which a particular therapy is compared to an alternative such as a waiting list, usual care, or another treatment. Because it is difficult to design a research study involving very long-term therapy, most EBPs are short-term (20 sessions or less, usually over a period of less than six months). Most EBPs are learning-based psychotherapies in which skills are taught, practiced, and designed to be used by the patient beyond the course of therapy. In this way, EBPs can be seen as comparable to physical or occupational therapy, in which patients are seen on a short-term basis to address particular problems, the therapist takes the role of teacher or coach, and exercises are practiced between sessions until a predetermined goal is reached or progress plateaus. Home care teams often include rehabilitation specialists, so patients are familiar with this form of practice, which may make EBPs easier to introduce in this setting.

Lists of EBPs can be found on websites maintained by the American Psychological Association Division 12 (www.div12.org/psychological-treat ments/) and the Substance Abuse and Mental Health Services Administration (www.samhsa.gov/ebp-resource-center). These treatments have been developed and tested for mental health (e.g., depression, anxiety), behavioral medicine (e.g., pain, insomnia), and substance use problems (e.g., smoking cessation). A complete list of EBPs is too long to reproduce in this chapter, so we focus on the most commonly used EBPs for the most typical problems seen in older home care patients. It should be noted that most of these therapies have not been evaluated in the home, although many have been tested via web-based applications or tele-mental health, and some have not been tested very thoroughly with older adults.

EBPs can be performed by anyone with appropriate training, within the scope of their practice. In this chapter, we refer to MH providers, who traditionally include psychologists, social workers, and psychiatrists, but we have seen EBPs used successfully by occupational therapists, nurses, physicians, peer counselors, and others.

EBPs are not synonymous with manualized treatments. Like most MH providers, we do not always use manuals exactly as written. However, we do practice according to EBP principles, meaning that treatment is time-limited, most sessions involve learning, and most conclude with the assignment of between-session practice. A home-based provider may carry a therapy toolkit that includes an assortment of handouts (e.g., a list of pleasant activities), worksheets (e.g., a sleep diary), and props (e.g., finger traps for Acceptance and Commitment Therapy). Some providers may also carry a whiteboard to respond flexibly in the session, just as in the office. It can be stimulating to develop one's own materials, sometimes using ideas generated by patients, rather than constraining oneself to do or use something that may not fit the situation or the patient because "It's in the manual for session 3."

Supportive therapy, although widely practiced in the office and in the home, is not typically considered an empirically-based psychotherapy, despite the fact that it is superior to waiting list and other no-treatment or minimal-treatment conditions. The main arguments in favor of supportive therapy for home care patients are that individuals seen in their homes are often socially isolated and therefore benefit most from social contact; due to physical or cognitive limitations they are not able to benefit from a learning-based therapy; they prefer supportive therapy to treatments that are structured and require work between sessions; and home care workload constraints preclude seeing patients on a sufficiently frequent basis to conduct EBPs. The counterarguments include evidence that EBPs have more powerful, rapid, and durable effects than supportive therapy, even with cognitively or medically compromised older adults; individuals seen in the home ought to have access to the best available treatments; it is our job to present patients with a menu of effective, feasible treatment options, which may not include everything the client could possibly want; and patients retain the autonomy to accept or refuse the services offered. From a practice-management perspective, providing supportive therapy frequently enough to make a difference to any one patient can limit the number of other patients a home-based MH provider can treat. For these reasons, we encourage all home-based MH providers to use EBPs as much as possible.

Why Conduct EBPs in the Home?

In-home MH providers should conduct EBPs because they work better than alternatives to alleviate symptoms quickly and help patients make lasting behavioral changes. Most evidence for conducting MH interventions in the home with older adults focuses on treating depression (Markle-Reid & McAiney, 2016). One particular EBP, Problem-Solving Therapy (PST), has been established as highly effective for depressed older adults (Kirkham, Choi, & Seitz, 2016). It is equally effective in person in the home (Gellis & Bruce, 2010) and via telephone (Choi et al., 2014). Of particular relevance, *in-home PST has demonstrated effectiveness, relative to supportive psychotherapy, for cognitively impaired and disabled depressed geriatric patients* (Kiosses et al., 2015). PST is the first EBP that the VA has rolled out specifically for in-home MH providers (PST-HBPC). Training in PST for non-VA clinicians is available through the AIMS (Advancing Integrated Mental Health Solutions) Center at the University of Washington (https://aims.uw.edu/collaborative-care/behavioral-interventions/pro blem-solving-treatment/training).

Telephone or tele-mental health interventions are effective with older people with depression (behavioral activation: Egede et al., 2015; PST: Choi et al., 2014); generalized anxiety (cognitive behavioral therapy, or CBT: Brenes, Danhauer, Lyles, Anderson, & Miller, 2017), fear of falling (CBT: Wetherell et al., 2018), and chronic pain (Acceptance and Commitment Therapy: Herbert et al., 2017).

In addition to their benefits for specific patients, EBPs can optimize the MH provider's overall practice. Careful practice management is critical because home care is such a limited resource, relative to clinic-based care. Some MH providers who work in the home respond to the pressure of large caseloads by making visits every month or every two months, with no a priori therapeutic endpoint. When new patients are added, visits to all patients become less frequent (and often the clinician feels more stress).

To date, research has not compared the efficacy of a short-term EBP delivered weekly or biweekly to a comparable number of visits spread out over the course of a year. Given what we know about human learning, it is reasonable to assume that skills are consolidated more effectively over a relatively short period of time. As therapists, it can be difficult remembering what practice exercises we discussed with patients last week without resorting to our notes; it is virtually impossible to imagine following up on "homework" assigned to an older adult two months ago. Therefore, infrequent sessions often means the therapy is not truly an EBP, despite the best intentions of the MH provider. With infrequent sessions, there may be some attempt to, for example, perform cognitive restructuring in the moment, but the odds are low that patients will internalize the skill to the point of being able to use it on their own to manage their mood.

Most importantly, virtually everyone would prefer to feel better in two months rather than two years. In consulting work, we have seen many cases of patients in treatment for eight to 10 years who report more improvement after eight weeks of an EBP than in the entire previous course of therapy. We owe it to these patients to alleviate their distress as quickly as we can, and then let them "graduate" rather than take on the permanent identity of a "mental health patient."

Who Isn't a Good Candidate for an EBP?

Some EBPs are appropriate for cognitively impaired patients, particularly if they have a caregiver who can serve as a coach or even perform the intervention. For example, caregivers can be taught to perform behavioral activation (pleasant activities scheduling) to alleviate depression in loved ones with dementia. The PST-HBPC protocol includes instruction on using caregivers as coaches. But because EBPs are learning-based interventions, patients who are unable to learn due to dementia or other cognitive disorders may not be good candidates for EBPs. For these patients, environmental adjustments, caregiver education, and pharmacotherapy are likely better choices than EBPs.

Other factors that temporarily detract from patients' ability to learn may make them poor candidates for EBPs. Individuals who are medically fragile, frequently hospitalized, or in transition between care settings (e.g., skilled nursing, rehabilitation) may need to wait until they are more stable to begin a course of EBP. Individuals in crisis (e.g., in the process of eviction or currently victimized by elder abuse) need to have their crisis addressed before they can learn new skills (which may help them avoid future crises).

How to Decide on an EBP

Although this is not unique to home-based MH care, the first challenge for a therapist planning to use an EBP is figuring out the target problem.

Most older adults receiving home care do not present with only one problem; a typical patient may have both depressive and anxiety symptoms, as well as cognitive impairment, inappropriate medication use, nonadherence to dietary recommendations, and conflict with an adult son or daughter. Although there is often no one right answer to the question "What should we work on (first)?" some issues merit consideration. First, prioritize anything that rises to the level of an emergency. This could be psychological (e.g., suicidal ideation), medical (e.g., smoking while on oxygen), or social (e.g., self-neglect). Second, consider whether a problem is likely to interfere with therapy; for example, focus on substance abuse issues first with a patient who is intoxicated during a visit. After considering these issues, take the patient's preferences into account. What is most distressing to the patient? It is often helpful to select the most severe or disabling problem that appears amenable to treatment. For example, a patient with panic attacks and hoarding disorder who would like to lose 20 pounds might benefit from starting with treatment for panic. Panic disorder is more disabling than being modestly overweight and is also more readily treatable than is hoarding. Successful treatment of panic symptoms is likely to increase the patient's motivation to work on weight or hoarding behavior.

Some patients have difficulty focusing on one issue. The MH provider may feel like therapy is a game of *Whac-A-Mole* with a new problem arising each week. It is most helpful in such cases for providers to avoid jumping from topic to topic and to model a rational problem-solving style in which one target is addressed until progress is made. The ability to gently and repeatedly redirect a patient is critical in these situations.

Some therapists have difficulty sticking to an agenda when a patient presents as highly distressed. It can be tempting to throw the EBP out the window and provide supportive listening when faced with a sobbing patient. Beware of that impulse – encouraging patients to work in therapy while accommodating the presence of negative emotions teaches them that they are stronger than their distress. Linking the upsetting precipitating event to in-session skill development and practice in therapy can be a respectful way of acknowledging the distress while gently helping the patient to move forward and make progress towards previously identified goals.

EBPs and Practice Management

It may seem obvious that the choice of an EBP should be guided by what works for the problem at hand, what the therapist can do, and what the patient prefers. Although patient preference is important, we believe that practice-management principles should also be considered before presenting options to a patient. Specifically, knowing how many appointment "slots" an MH provider has in a year, and dividing that by the number of patients the provider expects to see in a year for therapy, indicates the approximate number of sessions available to treat each patient.

If an MH provider knows that she has about six sessions, on average (including the initial visit in which the diagnosis is made and the care plan developed in collaboration with the patient), to help each new patient reduce symptoms or make behavioral changes, this is the starting point for the choice of intervention: *What would make the best possible use of the six sessions available to treat this patient?* The need for efficiency in this provider's practice would pull for an EBP even if she were trained in other models of psychotherapy.

Note that the number of sessions per patient also affects the way that the identified problem is defined. The patient may say that he suffers from low self-esteem and wants psychotherapy to address that problem. To our knowledge, there are no EBPs, let alone six-session EBPs, that specifically raise self-esteem. Because the focus of EBPs is on current problems, the therapist needs to quickly help the patient translate low self-esteem into particular emotional or behavioral symptoms that can reasonably be addressed in approximately six sessions. In this case, improving depressed mood and reducing isolation are appropriate targets for intervention. A patient who continues to report low self-esteem but is less depressed and more socially engaged after six to eight sessions would count as a success in this model of practice.

Other factors to consider when selecting an EBP are patient- or situation-specific. For example, the patient may be at a distance (100 miles) that makes only two in-person visits possible within a two-week period, with no visits for some period of time. (As described above, there is very limited evidence for the effectiveness of interventions conducted at longer intervals than two weeks.) The patient may not be cognitively or technologically equipped to use tele-mental health services. The patient may be hesitant to take a psychotropic medication. The provider thus has to select from a menu of interventions she knows she can conduct in two in-person sessions, based on the presenting problem; for example, behavioral activation for depression, relaxation training for anxiety, or motivational interviewing (MI) to increase willingness to accept a psychotropic medication.

The MH provider must also assess factors such as:

1   How acute is the patient's psychiatric illness? For example, is this someone who has made a recent suicide attempt? It may be that the focus of the provider's work must be helping the patient find an accessible source of MH treatment urgently, which would involve working closely with the team's social worker to establish links to community resources.
2   How strongly opposed to medication is the patient? Is it likely that two sessions of MI could bring the person past the precontemplation

or contemplation stage? If logistical factors preclude the possibility of an EBP (e.g., inability to schedule visits weekly or every other week for two to three months), medications may be the best available alternative.

3   What other team members are available to partner in MH care for this patient? For example, the team may include other members who have training in MI, supporting the MH provider in initiating this form of intervention. Other team members can also administer a brief self-report measure to help the MH provider track symptoms over time.

4   Does the patient have a caregiver who can be enlisted as a coach? As the old adage goes, "two heads are better than one" when it comes to learning and practicing a new skill, making the therapy process more efficient.

In this case, the provider makes a diagnosis of post-traumatic stress disorder (PTSD), assesses other relevant factors, determines that the patient is not in acute crisis and has low risk of suicide, and decides that the most desirable option is to teach the patient one relaxation strategy (a simplified form of progressive muscle relaxation) during the first session, leaving a recording to facilitate between-session practice. During the second session, she reviews the homework, teaches a second relaxation strategy (guided imagery), and provides information about PTSD and PTSD treatments, including medications, as appropriate for someone in the precontemplation stage. At the end of the second session, the MH provider leaves the patient with her contact information, arranges for a telephone check-in in one month, discusses with the social worker options for the patient to receive appropriate MH care close to home, lets the team members trained in MI know the status of the patient's current willingness to consider psychotropic medication, and asks the nurse who sees the patient every two months to administer the PTSD Checklist at every visit and keep the MH provider apprised of the results.

Introducing EBPs to a Home Care Patient

We find that it is actually quite easy to introduce the idea of an EBP to a patient receiving in-home services. The following is a transcript of a first visit with a new patient, a 74-year-old Chinese American woman with end stage renal disease. The first 45 minutes of the session consisted of an assessment during which the MH provider determined that the patient's primary problem was depression. At this point in a typical first visit, the task is to present feedback to the patient and collaborate on a treatment plan.

THERAPIST: So, Mrs. Lee, let me summarize what you've been telling me, just to make sure I have it right. You said that you have been feeling depressed for about the past four months, ever since you went on dialysis. You've been having trouble sleeping, your concentration hasn't been good, and you've been losing weight because you just don't feel like eating. Everything seems like an effort, and you feel like you're a burden to your family. You still enjoy calligraphy and spending time with your family, but you aren't doing either of those things very often. You remember feeling depressed like this in your forties during your divorce, and you saw a therapist for a couple of years at that time. You said you are not having any thoughts about harming yourself and you've never done anything to harm yourself in the past. Did I miss anything?

MRS. LEE: Well, all those things are true. I would never try to hurt or kill myself because that would cause my family so much pain. But my main problem is that I'm on dialysis. That means going to a center three days a week, almost all day, and feeling exhausted most of the time even on days when I'm not on dialysis. Wouldn't anyone feel depressed if they had to go through this?

THERAPIST: It's completely natural to feel bad when bad things happen, like your divorce back then and your kidney disease now. And being on dialysis is a problem. The thing is, if you also have depression, that's two problems. If there were a way for you to feel less depressed, that would be one less problem.

MRS. LEE: I would like to feel better, but I can't imagine that happening. I'm not a good candidate for a kidney transplant, so I will probably be on dialysis for the rest of my life.

THERAPIST: I understand your doubts, but are you willing to give working with me a try?

MRS. LEE: Are you going to start coming every month like my nurse does?

THERAPIST: I would actually like to come once a week for a couple of months, if that's alright with you, to help you learn some new skills so that you'll feel less depressed.

MRS. LEE: Are there skills for that? My other therapist just talked, or rather, mostly just listened. It was so helpful to get it all out.

THERAPIST: You said you saw her for a little over two years, right? How long did it take for you to feel better?

MRS. LEE: Well, I started seeing her after the divorce papers were filed, and I didn't start to feel better until about a year after the divorce was final. I think that's normal, though, don't you?

THERAPIST: A year is a long time to feel depressed. I don't want you to feel depressed for a year. I would like to see you feel at least a little better in a couple of months.

MRS. LEE: Do you think that's possible?

THERAPIST: Mrs. Lee, in my experience, even older people with serious medical conditions can feel less depressed if they learn and practice some strategies for managing their mood. I'm thinking there are three things we could work on, and I'd like your input in choosing one of them. The first option is to focus on what you're doing and how you're spending your time. You mentioned that everything's an effort, so you haven't been doing calligraphy or spending as much time with your family. And not doing things you enjoy means you aren't feeling much joy, which is one reason you're depressed. A second option is to explore some of the thoughts you're having that may not be helping you. You said you think feeling depressed is normal in your situation; I wonder if that means you think you will always be depressed from now on? When you think those thoughts, it probably makes you feel even worse. Finally, the third thing we could focus on is one of the problems you're facing. When you talk about dialysis, your main concern seems to be feeling exhausted a lot of the time. If we worked on the problem of fatigue, and made that even a little bit better, do you think you might feel less depressed?

MRS. LEE: That's a lot of choices. You said we could try to work on my fatigue, or on how I'm spending my time, or on what I'm thinking about?

THERAPIST: Yes, in my experience, any of those choices could help you feel at least a little better in a couple of months. But we should pick one, so we stay focused, and you and I will agree each week on some things you will do between sessions. I call it practice; some of my other patients call it homework.

MRS. LEE: I'm curious what "homework" for depression will be like! I don't understand how thinking has anything to do with dialysis. It sounds like magic to believe that I can think my way out of kidney disease. But I agree that if I could feel less tired on the days I don't have to go in for dialysis, things would be easier.

THERAPIST: Ok, then. We are going to start doing something called Problem-Solving Therapy. This type of treatment has helped many older people with depression, including those with serious medical problems like being on dialysis. We are almost at the end of our time today, but I'm going to give you a handout to read that describes some basic information about Problem-Solving Therapy, and then we can talk about it more next week. How does that sound?

MRS. LEE: Is that my "homework"? Reading this handout?

THERAPIST: You caught me! Yes, that's right. Are you willing to read it? And you can jot down questions or reactions so we can be sure to talk about them next time.

MRS. LEE: That sounds good. Will you come next Tuesday, then? Same time as this week? Tuesdays seem to be my best days right now.

THERAPIST: I will see you next Tuesday. It was a pleasure to meet you, Mrs. Lee, and I'm glad we'll be working together.

In this example, the therapist introduced the idea of a time-limited therapy process involving learning and between-session practice, in contrast to the patient's past experience with long-term supportive therapy. She offered the patient a choice between behavioral activation, cognitive restructuring, and PST, all EBPs for depression that the therapist deemed potentially appropriate for this patient, using language and examples drawn from the patient's description of her situation. She began building rapport and obtained buy-in to proceed with treatment, including the first homework assignment. She is well positioned to work with the patient on a six- to eight-session course of PST.

Challenges Conducting EBPs in the Home

EBPs can be interrupted by hospitalization, rehabilitation stays, transitions to skilled nursing facilities, and discharge from the home care service. In our experience, the fact that EBPs often involve handouts and other memory aids makes them easier to resume after an interruption. If therapy must be terminated altogether, the patient retains the materials and the knowledge to continue using skills previously taught. Caregivers or other supportive individuals who partner with the MH provider during therapy can also facilitate continued progress or maintenance of gains.

Will a home care patient accept an EBP? As stated above, EBPs can be compared to physical or occupational therapy, with which many home care patients have experience. Although some may have different expectations of psychotherapy, perhaps influenced by the media, the movies, or their past experience with outpatient MH care, in our experience they can and do understand an EBP practice model in the home. In fact, in our experience, many older patients who are skeptical about "shrinks" find the idea of working with a "coach" more acceptable.

Also as discussed above, most EBPs are based on a learning model and therefore require patients to practice skills between sessions. What to do about a patient who repeatedly does not engage in between-session activities? As is usually the case, the first step is diagnosis: What is the barrier? Does the patient understand and accept the idea that practice is necessary to learn new skills? All people have had experience with learning that required practice – sports, musical instruments, driving, bathing a baby – and finding the example or metaphor that resonates with that particular patient is the essence of the therapist's art. Does the patient understand the rationale for the particular exercise? A collaborative relationship between patient and therapist is every bit as important in EBPs as in supportive counseling or psychodynamic practice; perhaps more so. There are many ways of achieving most objectives and working together to design a practice exercise can be an example of creative joint problem-solving (which may have the additional benefit of fostering the working alliance between patient and therapist). Is the exercise too difficult? Deficits in memory, vision, hearing, strength, knowledge, time, finances, and other resources can all interfere with the ability to carry out even the best intentions. Here, being in the patient's home is a huge advantage. We can often guide the patient in practicing the exercise the first time while we are present; this also helps spot potential roadblocks (e.g., it may not be realistic for an older patient who wants to get more exercise but lives on a steep hill to go out for daily walks in the neighborhood) that we can problem-solve with the patient. We can help the patient find or place cues in the environment to remember practice exercises, like posting a note on the bathroom mirror. And we can see first-hand when a task needs to be broken down. An outpatient therapist may endorse a patient's plan to clean house, whereas a therapist in the home of someone with hoarding disorder knows that the process will be slow and difficult.

What if patients are not interested in an EBP? Sometimes all this means is that the patient refuses to do written "homework." Between-session learning and practice should always be adapted to the particular needs of the patient, meaning that not all homework has to be written. Some patients, however, are not interested in learning at all and "just want to talk." As is true for all healthcare professionals, we must accept that our patients have the right to refuse any service; in turn, they must accept that *we are not going to provide all possible services*, especially if we do not have the resources. The physical therapists on our teams will not allow for endless sessions if patients are willing to exercise with them but not independently between visits. Our physical therapists also do not have time to visit patients, even those with physical disabilities or high fall risk, monthly or bimonthly on a long-term basis. Sometimes other team members who see the role of the MH provider as mainly offering social support may need these explanations as well.

It is possible to conduct one or two sessions of MI with patients to discuss the advantages and disadvantages of engaging in an EBP; for those patients who remain in the precontemplation or contemplation stage regarding a treatment that is based on learning skills and requires between-session practice, we leave our contact information and offer to see the patient again in the future if motivation changes. The provider remains available for crisis management at the request of the team, patient, or caregiver, but we do not typically set a routine schedule of in-person visits every so often to "check in." (And the fact that we do not perform regular "check-in" visits for numerous long-term patients gives the time and flexibility in our schedules to see patients who are in crisis more easily, and to see psychotherapy patients weekly to conduct EBPs).

MH providers who are working on a team can and should collaborate with other disciplines involved in a given patient's care. On our teams, nurses usually see patients on a schedule ranging from every two weeks to monthly. It is easy to ask a nurse to give a patient a depression questionnaire such as the Patient Health Questionnaire-9 at every visit; elevated scores can then trigger initiation or re-initiation of MH services.

This eliminates much of the need for "check-in" visits by the MH provider. Nurses can also be taught basic empathic listening skills (some are quite adept already) and can sometimes plan to schedule an extra 15 minutes into a visit for supportive contact with a patient who "just wants to talk" (some do this anyway). They can also learn enough about therapy techniques such as behavioral activation to prompt continued practice.

Sometimes the barrier to conducting EBPs lies within ourselves. For example, during consultation, a therapist stated that she didn't feel comfortable engaging in role plays with patients because it felt "too infantilizing." With further discussion, it emerged that her own social anxiety made role plays extremely uncomfortable for her, and she projected that discomfort onto patients. After more discussion, she decided to disclose her own anxiety to facilitate rapport with a patient who could benefit from practicing a difficult conversation with a family member. As it turned out, both therapist and patient had a very successful experience during the role play, and the patient subsequently carried out the conversation as practiced, with a positive outcome. In turn, the exposure lessened the therapist's anxiety about conducting role plays with future patients.

Some MH providers are skeptical of EBPs. (We assume that people who choose to read this chapter may be skeptical but not totally resistant.) Dr. Marsha Linehan, the developer of Dialectical Behavior Therapy, used to speak about how much more enjoyable it is for therapists to have "heart-to-hearts" with patients than to conduct less pleasant elements of EBPs such as setting an agenda, maintaining structure within the session, keeping time, redirecting patients, assigning and checking up on between-session practice, etc. An MH provider in the process of being trained in an EBP would repeatedly say to one of us, "If I were doing *real* therapy, I would do such-and-such." For therapists who do not have much faith in EBPs to begin with, it is easy to find reasons not to do them in the home.

Case Examples

We have found through years of training other MH providers to perform EBPs in the home that one of the best ways to increase motivation is to see them work. In this spirit, we present two examples of patients we've treated using EBPs in the home.

Insomnia: Mr. Cross

Mr. Cross was an 87-year-old Black man. He lived with his wife, who identified herself as his primary caregiver. Mr. Cross's medical conditions included macular degeneration, hearing loss, and hypertension. Performance on a brief screening test suggested intact cognition. Personal psychiatric history was negative, although at the time of the home care MH provider's assessment, he reported significantly impaired sleep. Mr. Cross described frequent nighttime awakenings with difficulty reinitiating sleep. He shared that he had not slept at all one night in the previous week. Although he indicated that he had always been a "light sleeper," the degree of sleep difficulties was unusual for him. His wife noted significant daytime fatigue. They could not identify any particular triggers to his sleep disturbances and reported these changes had been present for about two to three months. Mr. Cross indicated interest in nonpharmacological interventions for insomnia and, with his permission, his wife agreed to be involved in his treatment.

The MH provider met weekly with Mr. and Mrs. Cross in their home over the course of eight sessions. Treatment was a form of CBT for insomnia (CBT-I) that involved psychoeducation around sleep, including the importance of behavioral activation and the need to avoid naps during the day despite daytime somnolence. Mrs. Cross was crucial to implementation of the recommended interventions, as she helped keep Mr. Cross awake during the day and encouraged him to increase his activity level. She also helped remind him when he was engaging in habitual behaviors that were not conducive to sleep (e.g., listening to the news right before bedtime, which Mr. Cross found activating and anxiety-provoking). She completed a sleep diary for Mr. Cross, as he was unable to do so due to his visual impairments. Through this work, she and the patient were able to identify patterns and areas for improvement, including goals for sleep restriction.

Over the course of treatment, Mr. Cross continued to demonstrate some problematic behaviors that his wife had difficulty controlling. For example, despite increasing his daytime activity, he continued to nap during the day for 30–60 minutes. Given his advanced age and overall improvement in sleep efficiency and quality, reduction of naps was not a primary focus of treatment. After Mr. Cross reported consistently improved sleep and demonstrated good understanding and practice of recommended interventions, treatment was terminated. He described his sleep as "wonderfully improved." Mr. Cross has since reached out for "booster sessions" related to reviewing good sleep hygiene techniques, and both he and his wife appear to have benefitted from these occasional reminders.

Health Anxiety and Depression: Mr. Thomas

Mr. Thomas was a 69-year-old White widowed man who lived alone in low-income independent senior housing. He presented with significant chronic medical conditions, including congestive heart failure, atrial fibrillation, oxygen-dependent chronic obstructive pulmonary disorder, and Type II diabetes. His mobility was limited, requiring a wheelchair or scooter outside of his home. He lived on a fixed income with no personal transportation. His adult son and daughter lived in the area and provided help on request.

Mr. Thomas presented with moderate to severe anxiety related to his health conditions, and moderate depression related primarily to his loss of independence and associated lifestyle changes. A gregarious man who had found purpose serving as a lay minister at his church and a volunteer in a civic organization, he struggled with the loss of social connections and sense of meaning. His isolation and limited activity disposed him to increased rumination about his health. His healthcare team referred him because of his frequent calls with healthcare questions and concerns.

The MH provider felt Mr. Thomas would benefit from a brief PST treatment protocol, but as he lived two hours from her office, psychotherapy in the home was not feasible. However, Mr. Thomas expressed comfort using computers and was open to participating in therapy through tele-mental health. After an intake at Mr. Thomas's home, follow-up therapy sessions were conducted using a secure telehealth program accessible on his personal laptop. Educational material accompanying the PST program was provided during the intake via both paper handouts and a publicly available web course.

Therapy first introduced coping skills to clarify stress and relieve cognitive overload, such as talking with others, prayer, and journaling on his computer. Mr. Thomas felt this helped him to clarify that his main need currently was to "love himself" better as he is now, and care for himself within his current circumstances. To this end, the next session focused on enhancing self-awareness of emotional states, especially when he may be excessively ruminating about his health and identifying pleasurable activities to focus his attention for improved mood (e.g., taking his dog outside to play, listening to music).

Next, therapy involved a guided problem-solving strategy. Working towards his goal of "loving himself more," Mr. Thomas identified and implemented several solutions to reach this goal. He made continued use of his stress management skills above, and also devised ways to increase his social connectedness and sense of meaning. He strengthened his existing social connections (e.g., calling friends more frequently, connecting with other residents at the apartment's dog park, attending communal lunches), and allowed others to provide him with transportation to events, overcoming his fear of being a burden that had previously prevented him from accepting help. He also found a new purpose for his experience as a lay minister by reaching out and providing support to others in his apartment community. By the end of treatment, he was going out of his apartment every day, and leaving the area for a social activity at least once a week. His health-related anxiety and depressive symptoms had significantly improved.

Providing therapy by telehealth differed from therapy in the home in only a few ways. An initial in-person visit was still critical to understanding Mr. Thomas's home environment and neighborhood. During that visit, educational materials for therapy were provided in advance. Mild technical issues presented initial challenges. For example, audio was difficult for Mr. Thomas to hear due to mild hearing impairment; this was addressed by his using headphones for sessions. A user-friendly telehealth software program was essential – Mr. Thomas had only to click a link in an email and the session room opened for him automatically. These adaptations were critical to make the therapy a successful experience.

Summary

The cases presented here illustrate some general principles about conducting EBPs in the home. First, most MH and behavioral medicine issues that respond to psychotherapy can be treated effectively in the home. Although the cases here focus on depression, health anxiety, and insomnia, three of the most common issues we see in our home care practice with older adults, we have also successfully treated patients with myriad diverse problems including PTSD, panic disorder, caregiver stress, marital conflict, chronic pain, smoking cessation, and obesity. Beyond PST and CBT, we use mindfulness training, Acceptance and Commitment

Therapy, and Interpersonal Therapy on a regular basis, and we have also used Prolonged Exposure, life review, integrative behavioral couples therapy, and stimulus control, among many other EBPs, with our home care patients. In our experience, any type of treatment that can be conducted in the office can be adapted for use in the home, and some (such as exposure therapy with *in vivo* behavioral practice) vastly more successfully.

Second, only one of these patients, Mr. Cross, had a fairly contained and clear problem. Mr. Thomas, with low income and very limited mobility, had moderate to severe anxiety, depression, and problematic behaviors that were interfering with his relationship with his healthcare team (repeated telephone calls seeking reassurance). MH providers are able to collaborate with complicated human beings with complex medical and MH issues to decide upon a primary focus for treatment and use EBPs to alleviate their distress.

Third, EBPs may be performed according to a manual, such as Mr. Thomas's PST intervention, or more flexibly as needed. It may be time for our field to replace "evidence-based psychotherapy" with "evidence-based practice," as this would more accurately reflect the work of most MH providers who use EBPs. The key EBP principles of learning and practicing new skills to focus on current problems in a time-limited format remain salient regardless of whether a specific manual is used.

Fourth, Mr. Cross's case suggests the utility of involving caregivers or supportive others in treatment. Sometimes this is essential, as when cognitive impairment interferes with the patient's ability to learn new skills. Sometimes it is convenient, as when a spouse who lives with the patient is accustomed to attending medical home care appointments. Of note, Mr. and Mrs. Cross had a collaborative, respectful relationship which appeared to enhance treatment efficacy. A caregiver-assisted EBP intervention would not likely be successful in couples with moderate to high conflict or personality variables related to oppositional reactions to suggestions and reminders.

Fifth, EBPs by telehealth need not be any less personalized than any other form of therapy. Personal connections and humor help strengthen rapport, as they do throughout the course of therapy in any modality. For example, the MH provider and Mr. Thomas met for a video session on Halloween in silly costumes. After Christmas, at the therapist's request, Mr. Thomas attended his therapy session in a giant furry hat his kids had given him – his favorite Christmas present. One of Mr. Thomas's main sources of emotional support was his Pomeranian, Ginger. Both Ginger and the therapist's dog, Barley, made occasional appearances on the webcam to greet one another and created a personal connection across the distance.

Throughout this chapter, we have assumed that our target audience is already experienced in conducting psychotherapy or other behavioral interventions with older adults. We further assume that they have received training in EBPs at some point in their careers but may find it hard to implement them in home care. We hope that this chapter will encourage MH providers who see patients in their homes to consider shifting their practice model away from check-in or supportive or "EBP-light" visits every six weeks to conducting EBPs in a manner that supports learning skills that linger after therapy is concluded. The former strategy "consumes" eight sessions per year per patient with slower symptomatic or behavioral progress; the latter will almost certainly yield greater improvement in a shorter amount of time while taking fewer sessions over the long term, thus enabling more home care patients to receive the benefits of psychotherapy.

References

Brenes, G. A., Danhauer, S. C., Lyles, M. F., Anderson, A., & Miller, M. E. (2017). Long-term effects of telephone-delivered psychotherapy for late-life GAD. *American Journal of Geriatric Psychiatry, 25*, 1249–1257.

Choi, N. G., Marti, C. N., Bruce, M. L., Hegel, M. T., Wilson, N. L., & Kunik, M. E. (2014). Six-month postintervention depression and disability outcomes of in-home telehealth problem-solving therapy for depressed, low-income homebound older adults. *Depression and Anxiety, 31*, 653–661.

Egede, L. E., Acierno, R., Knapp, R. G., Lejuez, C., Hernandez-Tejada, M., Payne, E. H., & Frueh, B. C. (2015). Psychotherapy for depression in older veterans via telemedicine: A randomized, open-label, non-inferiority trial. *The Lancet Psychiatry, 2*, 693–701.

Gellis, Z. D., & Bruce, M. L. (2010). Problem-solving therapy for subthreshold depression in home healthcare patients with cardiovascular disease. *American Journal of Geriatric Psychiatry, 18*, 464–474.

Herbert, M. S., Afari, N., Liu, L., Heppner, P., Rutledge, T., Williams, K., ... Wetherell, J. L. (2017). Telehealth versus in-person acceptance and commitment therapy for chronic pain: A randomized noninferiority trial. *Journal of Pain, 18*, 200–211.

Kiosses, D. N., Ravdin, L. D., Gross, J. J., Raue, P., Kotbi, N., & Alexopoulos, G. S. (2015). Problem adaptation therapy for older adults with major depression and cognitive impairment: A randomized clinical trial. *JAMA Psychiatry, 72*, 22–30.

Kirkham, J. G., Choi, N., & Seitz, D. P. (2016). Meta-analysis of problem-solving therapy for the treatment of major depressive disorder in older adults. *International Journal of Geriatric Psychiatry, 31*, 526–535.

Markle-Reid, M., & McAiney, C. (2016). Depression care management interventions for older adults with depression using home health services: Moving the field forward. *Journal of the American Geriatrics Society, 64*, 2193–2195.

Wetherell, J. L., Bower, E. S., Johnson, K., Chang, D. G., Ward, S. R., & Petkus, A. J. (2018). Integrated exposure therapy and exercise reduces fear of falling and avoidance in older adults: A randomized pilot study. *American Journal of Geriatric Psychiatry, 26*, 849–859.

13 Treating and Supporting the Caregiver

Angela W. Lau and Megan E. Gomez

'I lost my partner.' Mrs. Philips was devastated when her husband of 48 years had a stroke. 'He handled everything. I felt safe.' Now her husband required constant supervision and assistance with all of his care. Mrs. Philips had to learn how to care for him, how to be an advocate, and how to manage their finances and household by herself in the midst of grieving for the life she used to have. The couple have four children who are not involved in caregiving because 'they have families of their own.' Over the course of a year, Mrs. Philips lost almost 100 pounds. She started having piercing pain in her back and trouble walking, but she continued to provide all her husband's physical care because she did not want to place him out of the home.

****

'I'm a grown man, but I flinch every time she calls my name.' Mr. Klein's mother had an alcohol use disorder and was an emotionally and physically abusive parent. She has been diagnosed with Stage 4 breast cancer and can no longer take care of herself, but wants to die at home. Even though Mr. Klein resented his mother, he also felt sorry for her because she had alienated herself from everyone and was now all alone. Mr. Klein became his mother's caregiver. While she did show appreciation at times, Mr. Klein's mother continued to berate and denigrate him for everything he did. Mr. Klein was re-traumatized with each interaction, but he remained in his role because 'that's what she wanted.'

As the Baby Boomer generation ages, the number of people who may benefit from home-based care will continue to increase. Many people can live at home for many years with help from unpaid family and friends, and from paid community support. Informal caregivers play an increasingly vital role, taking on new roles and responsibilities, interfacing with healthcare and social service providers, and supporting their loved ones in being able to safely age in place.

The definition of a caregiver is a person who provides direct care to someone (Merriam-Webster Dictionary, 2016). In this chapter, we will be discussing caregiver issues for those who provide informal care to an older adult who requires help to function in his/her daily living.

Some do not like the word 'caregiver,' as it suggests a one-sided relationship. Other words for *caregiver* include *caretaker, care partner, carer*, or *guardian*. For the sake of consistency and ease of reading, we will refer to this role as 'caregiver' throughout this chapter, despite the limitations of the word. Similarly, we will use the term 'care recipient' (CR) to describe the person being cared for. Oftentimes, the term 'loved one' is used to identify the person being cared for, whether they are loved or not. By using the terms 'caregiver' and 'CR' we hope to minimize confusion about who is the identified patient.

Becoming a Caregiver

Mr. Wong knew his life partner had Alzheimer's disease. Over time, Mr. Wong started to take over doing the bills and managing their money. He became the contact person for his partner's doctors, and began to coordinate his medical care and manage his medications. Mr. Wong started taking over most of the household responsibilities because his partner started having trouble completing them.

****

Mrs. Taylor has become really worried for her parents. Her mom has Alzheimer's disease. In the past, her dad had been an excellent caregiver. Mrs. Taylor would only need to call periodically and go over on the weekends to help. As her dad became weaker and had memory problems of his own, Mrs. Taylor has slowly started calling her father during the day to remind him of things that needed to be done and helping with grocery shopping. Mrs. Taylor has also been taking more time off from work to attend her parents' medical appointments. More recently, her dad has fallen. He laughs it off, but Mrs. Taylor is afraid her parents need more care and supervision than she can provide. Mrs. Taylor is also experiencing guilt that she is not around enough for her two children, and that her husband must take on the bulk of their parenting and household responsibilities in addition to his full-time job. Mrs. Taylor isn't sleeping well and feels overwhelmed. She has been short-tempered and easily frustrated at work, at home, and with her parents. She feels like crying most of the time when she thinks about her responsibilities, and worries about how it will all get done.

One's ability to live independently is not always defined by what medical or psychiatric conditions one has, or even one's age, but rather how much a person can do for themselves. The caregiving role typically begins when the CR needs help with activities and tasks that need to be performed for independent living.

Activities of daily living (ADLs) include activities like basic self-care tasks, such as feeding, dressing, bathing, transferring (i.e., being able to get into and out of bed or chairs by oneself), toileting, and walking. Instrumental activities of daily living (IADLs) are still essential, but more complex, and include things like using the telephone, shopping for groceries, managing finances, meal preparation, housework, or laundry.

People become caregivers when they help the CR complete some or all of their ADLs and/or IADLs. The caregiver role may be assumed overnight if the CR experiences an acute injury and the CR becomes reliant on the caregiver's help in order to return to their own home (as opposed to being placed in an assisted living facility, board and care, medical foster home, or skilled nursing facility). In contrast, the process of becoming a caregiver may be gradual if the CR experiences slow declines in their functioning. The caregiver may eventually decide to move in with the CR or have the CR move in with them; either will be another major transition for both parties.

While family caregivers are normally a spouse, adult child, or another member of the immediate family, it is not uncommon for other people in the CR's life can step in and become caregivers, including non-blood relatives (e.g., in-laws, step-children), significant others, former spouses, kinfolk, close friends, or even acquaintances. It is important to identify who is serving in the role of a caregiver.

Joys of Being a Caregiver

In the book *The Inspired Caregiver: Finding Joy While Caring for Those You Love*, Tia Walker says 'to care for those who once cared for us is one of the highest honors' (Speers & Walker, 2013). Many find personal satisfaction in helping their 'loved one' stay in their home if that is where they want to be. For those who had a positive relationship with the CR, being their caregiver can enhance the emotional connection shared. Some cultures value caring for older adults and promoting their sense of dignity. Others value caring for the CR in the home where younger generations (e.g., grandchildren) can witness the commitment and devotion to the CR.

Challenges of Being a Caregiver

It is important to recognize that some caregivers may have concurrent caregiving responsibilities, including caring for their parents, children, or grandchildren, or another older adult relative. Many caregivers are also still working either part- or full-time. It can feel overwhelming to add caregiving to the list of competing responsibilities. Some caregivers may suffer financially from reducing their work hours or leaving the workforce entirely to provide the CR with the level of care needed. Caregivers may have to deal with the stress of potentially losing their jobs if their caregiving role is affecting their ability to be a productive employee.

Caregivers may also feel they do not have enough time for self-care. Many caregivers report problems attending to their own health and well-being while managing caregiving responsibilities. They report sleep deprivation, poor eating habits, failure to exercise, failure to stay in bed when ill, and postponement of or failure to make medical appointments for themselves (Shultz & Beach, 1999).

Caregivers may also feel a deep sense of inadequacy and frustration when interfacing with medical institutions, insurance companies, medical providers, and other ancillary services or community agencies. Many caregivers do not have a medical background, and health literacy may be low. They may experience pressure to demonstrate a very steep learning curve to function at the level their CR needs them to perform.

If the caregiver is caring for a person with challenging behaviors (e.g., agitation, non-adherence) or someone who does not do well in the CR role, it can seem impossible to get the CR to be adherent to the treatment recommendations, such as changing eating habits, taking medications as prescribed, and cooperating with bathing/hygiene.

Assessing Caregiver Burden

Clinical Interviews

A thorough clinical interview with a caregiver will aid in better understanding their roles/responsibilities, current symptoms of caregiver stress, history of caregiving for the CR, and history of past caregiving for others. Important elements of the interview include:

- The relational history between the caregiver and CR.
- What support system the caregiver has (perceived and actual).

- Available assistance and resources for the caregiver.
- How much respite they have in place, and other stressors/responsibilities that exacerbate caregiver stress.
- How they cope with stress and manage self-care.
- Their knowledge of the CR's condition(s), medical literacy.
- Their health beliefs, cultural values, spiritual beliefs, and expectations for caregiving or for people who need help.
- Their treatment goals.

Standardized Self-Report Measures

Self-report questionnaires can be used to supplement a clinical interview to identify caregiver stress. It can also be used to assess change throughout the course of treatment. The four-item Zarit Burden Interview-Screening Form and 12-item Zarit Burden Interview-Short Form (Bedard et al., 2001), and the 18-item Caregiver Self-Assessment Questionnaire (developed by the American Medical Association) are commonly used and easily administered in the home setting. Some caregivers may under-report stress for various reasons. Ethnic minorities, for example, may under-report symptoms due to cultural factors (Aranda & Knight, 1997). As such, it is important to gather qualitative data on caregivers and not solely rely on their endorsement of symptoms.

Collateral Information

It can be extremely helpful to hear about any observations or concerns regarding the caregiver from other team members, family members, and even from the CR if they are cognitively intact.

Benefits of Psychotherapy for the Caregiver

Reducing Caregiver Stress

Caregiver stress can lead to depression, anxiety, sleep disturbance, changes in appetite, low frustration tolerance, memory and other cognitive issues, withdrawal/isolation, and physical illness (Shultz & Beach, 1999). As caregiver stress escalates, it can interfere with the caregiver's ability to effectively perform their caregiving duties or to provide an optimal quality of life for the CR. Caregivers may forego their own physical and emotional needs and prioritize the needs of the CR. However, this can lead to the caregiver becoming so ill they can no longer provide care to the CR.

Individual or family psychotherapy can be very helpful if the burdens of being a family caregiver start to negatively affect the caregiver's physical and mental health. Psychotherapy and health/behavior interventions can be very effective in helping the caregiver better cope with the caregiving role, so they can provide optimal care and quality of life to the CR safely and for as long as possible in their home. By improving caregiver outcomes (reducing caregiver stress and decreasing burdens, anxiety, depression, and frustrations), we can, in turn, improve CR outcomes.

Programs such as Resources for Enhancing Alzheimer's Caregiver Health (REACH), REACH II (designed to better meet the needs of culturally diverse caregivers), and the Stress-Busting Program have been found to improve caregiver well-being and have been widely and successfully disseminated through health systems nationwide at the federal, state, and local levels. Similar online workshops, such as Building Better Caregivers (based on the eponymous book), are available to build skills and confidence for caregivers (Lorig et al., 2018). There are also caregiver support lines and informal peer support mentoring programs.

Preventing Caregiver Burnout

'I'm done ... I can't do it anymore.' Left untreated or allowed to escalate, caregiver stress can become caregiver burnout. This is when a caregiver can no longer tolerate the emotional stress and physical exhaustion that comes with their caregiver role and responsibilities (Almberg, Grafstrom, & Winblad, 1997). Caregivers experiencing caregiver burnout may want to quit their caregiver role, feel unable to provide optimal care to the CR, and/or feel unable to maintain quality of life for their CR. Treatment goals may include:

* Psychoeducation on caregiver stress, stress management, and effective problem-solving.
* Skills training, education on CR's health conditions, improving health literacy and self-efficacy.
* Identification of barriers in the caregiving experience (e.g., maladaptive thoughts).
* Increasing social, emotional, and physical support to reduce caregiver burden.
* Education on community services and programs (i.e., adult day health centers, in-home caregivers, meals on wheels, respite stays).
* Improving communication between caregiver and CR, other paid caregivers, and medical team.
* The importance of and permission to engage in self-care to reduce caregiver stress (Gallagher-Thompson & Coon, 2007; Gallagher-Thompson et al., 2003; Lewis et al., 2009).
* Mood and anxiety management strategies.
* Discussion of when placement to a higher level of care will be needed.

Psychoeducation and Behavior Management

Mr. Wong knew not to get upset when his partner repeated himself or asked the same question over again. But Mr. Wong couldn't help getting frustrated with his partner for not helping around the house anymore unless Mr. Wong asked him to do a specific chore. Frustration turned into exasperation when Mr. Wong's partner did not complete the task even after he agreed. Mr. Wong felt like his partner was not appreciating all that Mr. Wong already had to do for him and around the house. Mr. Wong perceived his partner was not being helpful or considerate enough of their situation.

Caregivers providing care to a person with Major Neurocognitive Disorder (MNCD), formerly known as dementia, may not have adequate knowledge of what MNCD is, its progressive nature, possible behavioral/personality changes, and what to expect. Without this knowledge, the CR's behaviors can evoke feelings of confusion, anxiety, frustration, anger, and/or sadness in the caregiver. The changing nature of the CR's personality, behaviors, and functioning can be especially challenging for family caregivers to try to understand and manage.

Providing psychoeducation about MNCD to normalize behaviors and reduce any unrealistic expectations that might cause frustration and other negative reactions by a caregiver can be important. Learning to identify the 'ABCs' (antecedent–behavior–consequence) of behavior and coaching the caregiver to develop effective behavior management strategies to address their CR's challenging behaviors can help instill understanding and compassion.

Mr. Wong was provided with psychoeducation on the progressive nature of MNCD and learned how to do a behavioral analysis (ABCs) so he could develop behavioral and environmental management strategies to help address some of his partner's more challenging behaviors. Mr. Wong was also referred to the local Alzheimer's Association chapter for ongoing caregiver support as his partner's condition advanced. With his new tools, Mr. Wong was able to better cope with and develop strategies for managing and preventing his partner's challenging behaviors.

Addressing Relational Dynamics

Providers may assume that the caregiver and CR had a neutral or positive relationship before the CR needed more assistance and supervision. Spouses may have been living together in a high-conflict relationship or leading separate lives before one partner became disabled. An adult child may have experienced a parent as absent, overly critical, playing favorites with their other siblings, or just mismatched in personality and temperament while growing up. Sometimes the caregiver makes the conscious choice to take on this role for their estranged or abusive family member. However, at other times the caregiver is a hesitant participant in the CR's care, and is only providing care out of obligation, duress, or fear of legal or financial consequences (e.g., they need the person's income to remain housed, there are no other next of kin to take the role).

Treatment would focus on helping to validate and support the caregiver's experiences, helping them develop ways to cope with challenging emotional experiences (trauma, ingrained negative relational dynamics) that can exacerbate baseline caregiver stress. If the CR is relatively cognitively intact, conjoint sessions may be an option to try to establish more effective communication patterns, and to create a more psychologically safe and reinforcing environment.

Mr. Klein greatly benefited from having someone listen, acknowledge, and validate his emotionally wrought situation. In treatment, he was able to identify the values that led him to his current predicament and, in turn, to suffer less when recognizing he made a value-based decision to be his mother's caregiver. He was able to work through some of his trauma reactions, manage anxiety, and increase self-care activities to improve his distress tolerance. Mr. Klein was able to identify and assert better boundaries when interacting with his mother to reduce his feelings of vulnerability and worthlessness. He was able to increase his self-esteem and self-efficacy and optimize the quality of care he provided to his mother.

Patient–Caregiver Conflict Related to Role Reversal

Some CRs that base their identity on being self-sufficient and autonomous may struggle with relinquishing control to a spouse or child when they are used to being in charge and making their own decisions. When an adult child, grandchild, or other relative from a younger generation becomes the caregiver, they may experience resistance and opposition from the CR due to the CR having a hard time with the role reversals that have resulted from someone younger having control or supervising them. Frequent complaints include feeling that the caregiver is being disrespectful and/or treating the CR 'like a child.' 'I used to be the parent, and now I'm the child.' Similarly, a CR husband from a more patriarchal marriage may have difficulty having a caregiver wife 'tell me what to do' and 'try to control me.'

Treatment would focus on helping the caregiver manage the anxiety they feel to 'do what's right' for their CR and the frustration and anger they may feel when the CR 'won't listen to me' or 'is fighting me' by helping the caregiver take an empathetic stance and accept their role as the advocate for the CR's patient-identified goals (or pre-identified wishes if they no longer have capacity). It could also include teaching the caregiver how to engage in motivational interviewing with their CR, working on how to communicate or present information to the CR and how to problem-solve and negotiate the line between prioritizing safety against respecting the CR's autonomy.

Improving the Working Relationship between the Caregiver and Treatment Providers

Since the caregiver is oftentimes the point person and/or decision-maker for the CR, it is critical that the provider–patient relationship, now the provider–caregiver relationship, is strong and collaborative. Unfortunately, for a variety of reasons, caregivers may have difficulty working well with their CR's treatment providers.

Treatment could include helping caregivers identify the etiology of the conflict and helping to change the caregiver's perspective and behaviors in order to improve the working relationship between the caregiver and the provider(s). If the identified provider is part of your treatment team, you can also offer to facilitate joint sessions with the caregiver and the treatment provider to help identify points of conflict, facilitate conflict resolution, and help to develop a new pathway to foster and maintain a productive working relationship.

Identifying Goals of Care and Developing Treatment Plans

'I'm so mad at him.' Mr. Silva's doctor wants him to insert a G-tube now while his airway is still strong enough to undergo anesthesia, but he does not want any heroic measures or invasive procedures. Mrs. Silva has convinced her husband to get the G-tube because they still have school-aged children and 'We're not ready to let him go.' She can't understand why Mr. Silva keeps cancelling the pre-surgery appointments. 'He should just get the G-tube now in case he changes his mind later.' She has been having trouble sleeping and concentrating on tasks because she keeps focusing on the closing window for Mr. Silva to get a G-tube.

Mental health providers working in home care often help facilitate agreements of goals of care between CR and caregiver. When there is discord between the caregiver's goals and the goals of the CR, the provider can help close this gap. They can also help facilitate agreements of goals of care between the family and home care team. Often, these agreements are fluid and require revisions as conditions change (e.g., higher level of care, placement, invasive/aggressive intervention, palliative and/or hospice care).

Addressing Anticipatory Grief/Bereavement

For many caregivers, the road to saying goodbye to their CR is a slow and gradual one. With the CR's ongoing loss of functioning, the caregiver loses more and more of the former person they were married to, parented by, or befriended. At other times, the caregiver had their role traumatically thrust upon them when their CR had a sudden medical event that left the CR significantly disabled. Caregivers might have difficulty saying goodbye to the person they once knew, the life they once had, and the life they expected to have. Their fear, anxiety, and overwhelming sadness can interfere with the caregiver's ability to cope with their caregiving role, and facilitate caregiver burnout. Treatment might focus on providing the opportunity for the caregiver to grieve for their losses and come to a place of acceptance.

Mrs. Philips benefited greatly from an opportunity to grieve for her losses and to identify and process some of her catastrophic fears that prevented her from engaging in self-care when she had respite opportunities. She benefited from breathing retraining, worry containment, and mindfulness exercises so she could engage in stress reduction while engaging in caregiving responsibilities. She benefited from social skills training and role plays to ask for more help from her children. Mrs. Philips started to schedule short periods of time when she could meet with her friends or do something she enjoyed. She was able to stop worrying all the time and not feel so frustrated and sad when she provided care to her husband. She stopped putting off her own medical appointments and was able to get some procedures that helped reduce her pain.

Practical Considerations

Privacy

Privacy may be difficult to secure when meeting in the home setting because the CR is likely to be home at the time of the session with the caregiver. Trying to find a location within the home that is far enough away from the CR that the therapy session cannot be overheard, and yet close enough for the caregiver to still be able to provide supervision for the CR, can be tricky. Possible solutions include meeting out of the CR's earshot (e.g., in a backyard) or outside the home (a local park or establishment) if it can be arranged for someone to be in the home with the CR during your scheduled appointment with the caregiver. It is important to review any possible concerns over the lack of privacy if meeting in a public space or in any outdoor space where conversations can be overheard. However, it is up to the caregiver to make an informed choice given the cost/benefit of meeting outside the home setting.

Interruptions/Distractions

There may be interruptions from the CR (e.g., needing attention or ADL assistance) or by the responsibilities of a caregiver's role (e.g., telephone calls from providers, a paid caregiver has a question, other home agency visits). It can be extremely helpful to prepare for extra time to account for interruptions, scheduling a time with the caregiver when interruptions are least likely, or opting to meet when another person can be scheduled to provide the caregiver with respite time so they can focus on their session with you.

English may not be the preferred language for caregivers, or they may not speak English at all. If you are not competent in the caregiver's spoken language, then accommodations will need to be made. If the CR or another family member is the designated interpreter/translator for the caregiver, then there can be concern about whether the caregiver is being completely truthful during an assessment given lack of privacy.

If an interpreter is not available and the caregiver can speak and understand some English, moving forward with services can be strained because the caregiver may not be able to accurately and fully express their or her thoughts and feelings if speaking in English, or may not fully understand what you are trying to say to them or her.

Seeing if your practice or agency has access to a telephone interpreter/ translation service you can call into during a session can be helpful when providing home-based care. While using a professional interpreter/translator is always preferred, if you are working with a treatment team, as a last resort you can see if any other member of your team is fluent in the caregiver's language and is willing and able to serve as your interpreter/translator. It may also be prudent and valuable to research local cultural communities who may offer psychoeducational resources, individual therapy, or a support group in the person's preferred language.

Multiple Stakeholders

Some CRs will not have one primary caregiver, but rather a system of family members who, together, commit to ensure the CR's care needs are taken care of. As such, the primary caregiver may not be the designated decision-maker, whether formally (e.g., durable power of attorney) or informally (e.g., an adult child, instead of the spouse, makes the decisions).

Some families may have multiple decision-makers, and as such it may be difficult to implement some interventions (e.g., getting respite, behavior management strategies) because your caregiver does not have ultimate decision-making authority, or there are differences of opinions between the primary caregiver and other family members who provide some level of support.

Other Clinical Considerations

Supporting Your Team

In many instances, the home care team will spend most of their time working with the CR's family. The team may face challenges if there are several caregivers without one primary point person, dysfunctional family dynamics, or caregivers who are perceived by the team to be demanding, disrespectful, suspicious, or argumentative.

It is important to help the team members understand any dysfunctional dynamics so that changes can be made to develop a more collaborative working relationship. You can provide emotional support and suggestions on how team members can cope with caregivers with personality or psychiatric issues. Providing suggestions on how to effectively maneuver a complicated family system or not get into a power struggle with a challenging caregiver can only help improve the access and level of care the team has to the CR.

Advocacy

It may be difficult, but the MH provider may need to be an advocate for the primary caregiver if they are the surrogate decision-maker and there is a disagreement between the caregiver and the team regarding goals of care or a plan of care. The team would benefit from reminders to focus on developing patient-centered goals, the caregiver's right and responsibility to make decisions (if the CR does not have decision-making capacity or relinquishes decision-making to the caregiver), and to help team members identify and work through the anxiety and frustration they may feel when they can't optimize the CR's care and meet the goals they think are better for the CR.

Impaired Caregiver

What do you do if you suspect the caregiver has MNCD or other cognitive issues that are interfering with their ability to provide care to the CR? You would want to consider if it is really a neurocognitive disorder or maybe the caregiver is experiencing some cognitive inefficiencies due to the negative effects of stress, lack of sleep, and/or poor mood. It would be appropriate to refer the caregiver to his/her primary care provider for an evaluation to rule out any reversible conditions or identify any conditions that may be causing their cognitive impairment. If the cognitive impairment is causing significant dysfunction, you can try to get in touch with other family members to see if they share your concerns, rally support for the caregiver seeking medical attention, or for them to become more involved in and assist with the caregiver's responsibilities for the CR.

Summary

Each time we board a plane we hear the scripted details of how to first put on your own oxygen mask before you assist anyone else. Obviously, this is because before we can effectively help others we must first ensure our own safety. Caring for oneself is one of the most important yet often the most difficult thing a caregiver can do. By providing care to the caregiver, we can help the caregiver persevere and hopefully experience some meaning and joy in the marathon that is caring for a home-bound family member.

References

Almberg, B., Grafstrom, M., & Winblad, B. (1997). Caring for a demented elderly person – Burden and burnout among caregiving relatives. *Journal of Advanced Nursing, 25*, 109–116. doi:10.1046/j.1365-2648.1997.1997025109.x.

Aranda, M., & Knight, B. (1997). The influence of ethnicity and culture on the caregiver stress and coping process: A sociocultural review and analysis. *The Gerontologist, 37*, 342–354. doi:10.1093/geront/37.3.342.

Bedard, M., Molloy, D., Squire, L., Dubois, S., Lever, J., & O'Donnell, M. (2001). The Zarit Burden Interview: A new short version and screening version. *The Gerontologist, 41*, 652–657. doi:10.1093/geront/41.5.652.

Gallagher-Thompson, D., & Coon, D. W. (2007). Evidence-based psychological treatments for distress in family caregivers of older adults. *Psychology and Aging, 22*, 37–51. doi:10.1037/0882-7974.22.1.37.

Gallagher-Thompson, D., Coon, D. W., Solano, N., Ambler, C., Rabinowitz, Y., & Thompson, L. W. (2003). Change in indices of distress among Latino and Anglo female caregivers of elderly relatives with dementia: Site-specific results from the REACH national collaborative study. *The Gerontologist, 43*, 580–591. doi:10.1093/geront/43.4.580.

Lewis, S. L., Miner-Williams, D., Novian, A., Escamilla, M. L., Blackwell, P. H., & Kretzschmar, J. H. (2009). A stress-busting program for family caregivers. *Rehabilitation Nursing, 34*, 151–159.

Lorig, K., Laurent, D., Schreiber, R., Gecht-Silver, M., Gallager-Thompson, D., Minor, M., ... Lee, D. (2018). *Building better caregivers: A family caregiver's guide to reducing stress and staying healthy.* Boulder, CO: Bull Publishing Company.

Merriam-Webster Dictionary. (2016). *Definition of caregiver.* Springfield, MA: Merriam-Webster.

Shultz, R., & Beach, S. (1999). Caregiving as a risk for mortality: The caregiver health effects study. *Journal of American Medical Association, 282,* 2215–2219. doi:10.1001/jama.282.23.2215.

Speers, P., & Walker, T. (2013). *The inspired caregiver: Finding joy while caring for those you love.* Monterey, CA: Flowspirations LLC. CreateSpace Independent Publishing Platform.

14 Training Future Home-Based Care Providers

*Pamela L. Steadman-Wood and
Rachel L. Rodriguez*

Eric Richards is excited to be starting his clinical psychology predoctoral internship. He has always been interested in working with older adults and individuals with chronic illness. He was excited when his training director described a training experience that serves older adults with life-limiting illness. However, Eric was not expecting that he would have to travel to these patients' homes. He has so many questions: Will his supervisor be in the house with him for every session? Should he sit at the kitchen table or in the living room? Does he need to bring his own chair? What does he do if the patient has a medical emergency when he is in the house? Eric is feeling overwhelmed and not sure this will be a good fit, but is also eager to see how mental health (MH) care can be provided in the home setting.

Home care provides an exciting and unique opportunity for training MH providers at every stage of professional development, from practicum student to post-licensure professional. In fact, within one setting, occasions can arise for training in interdisciplinary, integrated teams (e.g., American Psychological Association, or APA, 2008), primary care (APA, 2015; McDaniel et al., 2014), geropsychology (APA, 2014; Knight, Karel, Hinrichsen, Qualls, & Duffy, 2009), health psychology (Larkin & Klonoff, 2014), rehabilitation psychology (Stiers et al., 2012), rural settings (Riding-Malon & Werth, Jr., 2014), and social work and other related areas of professional practice (Reckrey et al., 2014). However, with this diversity of training experiences come myriad considerations for preparing the trainee to practice, providing supervision, and evaluating competencies. This chapter will first evaluate these considerations at the pre-licensure level (e.g., practicum, master, predoctoral, postdoctoral) then delve into mentoring post-licensure professionals new to the home care setting. It will end with a discussion of interprofessional competency and the role of the MH provider in interdisciplinary team training.

Licensing Boards and Organizational Policies

One of the first steps in organizing a training experience in a home care setting is to review your state's professional licensing regulations for supervision. This will provide guidelines for supervision for the trainee. While many states do not stipulate the proximity of the trainee to the supervisor as services are being provided, some states do. For example, the state of Massachusetts prohibits a psychology trainee at any level from providing services unless the supervisor is present on the premises or in the immediate area. This means that the supervisor must accompany the trainee on all home visits where services are provided. If not, the trainee cannot count these as supervised hours for licensure in the state.

Next, it is important to review your organization's policies on the provision of home care, as this may also impact how and when the trainee can provide services. Field placements with private home care agencies will have orientation and training policies consistent with licensure laws and Medicare certification. This may (or may not) vary greatly from the practices in the public or government sector. In the VA (Veterans Affairs), there are clear guidelines regarding the proximity of the supervisor based upon the trainees' level of experience. A practicum student may not conduct independent home visits. The supervisor must always be physically present in the immediate area. Master's-level and predoctoral interns and postdoctoral fellows may make independent home visits provided that the supervisor is immediately available if consultation is needed. This consultation can be in person or via phone.

While the requirement that the supervisor must be physically present during home visits can appear to be a barrier to advanced training, there are creative solutions that will still allow the trainee to have an enjoyable and valuable learning experience. For example, if the patient lives in an assisted living facility or similar residence, the supervisor may be able to see a different patient in the facility at the same scheduled time. Or, if the patient's caregiver requires caregiver support or other intervention, the supervisor can provide these services in a different part of the home at the same time. A final suggestion is to have the supervisor located in another part of the home, or even in the car outside, where they can make telephone calls, write notes, or complete other professional tasks. Each of these suggestions will meet the requirement for the supervisor to be physically present for the trainee, while also allowing the trainee to meet with the patient independently.

A final point to consider is that your organization may also have guidelines regarding transportation to the patient's home. Trainees may need to undergo training to use the organization's car. Or they may be required to use their own vehicles. If the latter is the case, will the trainee receive reimbursement? If not, will that be a barrier for the trainee to completing home visits?

Orienting the Trainee to the Home Care Setting

Providing MH care in the home setting can be both an exciting and daunting concept to the new trainee. It is highly recommended that the trainee accompany the supervisor on several visits before making home visits alone; first, with the supervisor modeling the provision of services in the home, and then observing the trainee providing services. These joint visits can be crucial to easing the trainee into the home care setting, as well as allowing the supervisor to note any areas in need of further development in the trainee's practice prior to giving them more autonomy. Moreover, if you provide home care services as part of an interdisciplinary team, it is a great idea to have the trainee make joint visits with each discipline. This, again, can not only orient the trainee to service provision in the home, but can also provide valuable training on interdisciplinary team functioning.

Among the many important discussions to have with the trainee during the orientation is one regarding ethical considerations in home care. While many of these are discussed in other sections of this book, it is important to note them again here. Specifically, it is important to remind the trainee of ethical obligations related to confidentiality, multiple relationships, and informed consent and undue influence. Providing treatment in the home can make it difficult for the patient to refuse to participate in therapy, especially if the services are considered part of interdisciplinary team care. The patient may feel as though they "must" accept MH treatment or they cannot be part of the home care program. Additionally, cognitive impairment may make it difficult for the trainee to ascertain the patient's ability to consent to treatment. If the patient has a guardian or activated surrogate decision-maker, the trainee may need to reach out to that individual before beginning services with the patient. Privacy and confidentiality are always a challenge in home care. This includes not only additional individuals inside the home who may disrupt the therapy setting, but also individuals the trainee may meet on the way to the home. For example, one trainee arrived at the home at the same time as the postal worker who knew the patient very well. The postal worker asked many questions of the trainee, inquiring what services were to be provided to the patient, as well as providing valuable information about the patient's history. The trainee felt understandably uncomfortable but knew that it would be wrong to answer any questions. Encouraging the trainee to respond with a statement such as "I'm from [name of organization] and Mr. X is expecting me" may assist in such situation.

Perhaps one of the most difficult ethical considerations is that of multiple relationships. It is not uncommon for a patient to ask a provider for assistance with tasks that they cannot complete for themselves. For example, retrieving the mail for a patient who cannot walk to the end of their driveway where the mailbox is located may be reasonable and in the best interest of the patient's safety. However, picking up medications from a local pharmacy would constitute an alternate role. Hicken and Plowhead (2010) and Yang, Garis, Jackson, and McClure (2009) provide excellent overviews of these topics. The new trainee is often required to make on-the-spot ethical decisions in each of these areas, and it is important to not only prepare the trainee ahead of time, but also encourage the trainee to reach out to the supervisor if needed.

Creating a training manual is also recommended. It can contain valuable information regarding procedures and policies, documentation, and coding rubric, as well as a listing of contact information for key team members should the trainee need to contact an individual while in the field. Training manuals can also assist the trainee with crises or safety issues should they arise.

Preparing Trainees for Independent Home Visits

Once the trainee is oriented to the provision of MH services in the home, it is important to evaluate when they are ready for independent visits. Many training programs refer to this as graduated levels of responsibility. For the home care setting this not only requires the supervisor to evaluate adherence to the policies and procedures of home care, but also the trainee's overall clinical experience, judgment, knowledge, and technical skills as they relate to the ability to conduct services without the supervisor present.

While many of the following will likely also be covered during the orientation, it is important to review with the trainee important information to consider before meeting a patient for the first time:

1 What is the referral question?
2 What is the environment like? Are chairs and flat surfaces available? Any need to bring barriers to lay down before sitting?
3 Are there weapons in the home?
4 Is it a safe neighborhood? Any parking concerns? Any codes that are needed for entry?
5 Are there any pets that need to be put away before entering?
6 Are there other individuals that are usually in the home? Who can the provider talk to? Who else should be a source of information?
7 What are the patient's medical conditions? Medications?

    a Is there a need to consider infection control protocols?
    b Does the provider have hand sanitizer? A mask? Disposable gloves?

8 When should the trainee call 911 for a medical emergency?[*]
9 Does the patient have an advance directive and/or orders for life-sustaining treatments? Where is the paperwork located? Who is designated health care proxy?
10 If the patient is suicidal/homicidal or in need of psychiatric hospitalization, what is the protocol?[*]

The good news is that many of these questions can be answered by talking to the referral source and/or another team member if the trainee is part of an interprofessional team. Please also review Chapter 6 for additional safety concerns that MH providers must be aware of when working in the home care setting.

Interprofessional Competencies and Team Training

Patients receiving home care are often medically, psychologically, and socially complex. The patient may be receiving care from multiple providers and/or care from an interdisciplinary team. Chapter 2 provides an overview of the role of the MH provider in the interdisciplinary team setting, and the reader is encouraged to review it. However, the combination of interdisciplinary care and home care provides another distinctive opportunity for training that is worthy of brief discussion.

Kayla Burton is pursuing licensure in clinical social work and completing a field placement in a community home care agency. She had previous experience working in an outpatient MH clinic and worked with many patients with depression, anxiety, and substance use issues. At times, it can be difficult for the care team to understand all that she can offer to patients, and she feels as though her role is only to complete forms and find additional services. She knows that she can help her patients in more ways and is frustrated. She plans to talk with her supervisor about how she can expand her role.

Kayla's experience is not uncommon for many MH providers in an interdisciplinary team setting. Role expectations and role boundaries should be continually discussed and redefined. This is also important because significant overlap of roles and functions exists among MH professionals from varying training backgrounds. Encouraging your trainee to give short in-services during team meetings about MH services and appropriate referrals is not only an excellent opportunity to provide feedback on your trainee's teaching style but can also lead to a more satisfying training experience.

Dr. Amelia Tyler is completing a geropsychology postdoctoral fellowship in a VA medical center. She is completing a six-month rotation with the home-based primary care (HBPC) program. She enjoys working on the interdisciplinary team and is appreciative of the referrals. The team physical therapist, Walter, approached Amelia about a Veteran with whom he is having difficulty. The Veteran is a 75-year-old morbidly obese man who refuses to get out of bed and engage in physical therapy. He also has chronic back pain from a work-related injury which Walter believes is his main concern. Dr. Tyler scheduled a home visit and conducted an intake assessment with the Veteran. In addition to his chronic pain, the Veteran had many symptoms of anxiety and depression which also prohibited him from wanting to engage in physical therapy. Simply put, the Veteran feared that getting out of bed would result in falling and becoming more injured. They began a course of Cognitive Behavioral Therapy for chronic pain. Dr. Tyler and Walter conducted several joint home visits in which they were able to engage the Veteran in physical therapy exercises. She also met with Walter and reviewed relaxation and deep breathing techniques that he could use with the Veteran to address anxiety before engaging the Veteran in treatment.

From a training perspective, Dr. Tyler's experience shows how collaborative care can enhance both patient outcomes and team functioning. Important characteristics of functional collaborative care include the merging of expertise, division of labor, colleagueship, and distribution of power (Hinshaw, 1995). Trainees working on interdisciplinary teams are exposed to different disciplines' interpretations of patients' problems and approaches to problem-solving. Supervisors can help the trainee navigate these situations, demonstrating how the combined knowledge and skills that result from interprofessional collaboration will result in creative treatment approaches best meet the needs of the patient. The interdisciplinary team can also provide the supervisor with valuable feedback about the trainee's abilities. In short, training in interdisciplinary team functioning results in multilayered opportunities for supervision and evaluation.

Evaluating the Trainee

Evaluation is key to the training experience, and the home care setting necessitates that expectations for evaluation be clear from the start. Similar to traditional MH clinic settings, audio-recorded sessions can easily be done in the home with the use of digital recorders. However, video-recording of sessions may be more difficult as patients may not want images of their home taken. Either of these recording options will also require proper documentation of the patient's consent.

It is important that the supervisor relies on more than just the trainee's report of the MH intervention and patient progress. Therefore, it is strongly recommended that the supervisor set the expectation of multiple joint home visits throughout the course of the training experience. While the supervisor will make home visits with the trainee at the beginning of the experience for orientation and to determine the trainee's readiness to provide services independently, additional joint home visits can be scheduled at the mid-point and end of the rotation to evaluate the trainee's growth and skill. This *in vivo* supervision will likely increase trainee anxiety, but it is nonetheless key to evaluating their competence. In addition, if part of an interdisciplinary team, trainees may make occasional joint home visits with other disciplines. In this case, the team member can provide valuable feedback on trainee performance and interactions with the patient. Seeking feedback from the patient and/or their family can also provide a valuable source of information for evaluation.

Once the question of *how* to evaluate is answered, the next obvious question is *what* to evaluate. As noted at the beginning of this chapter, the home care setting provides a plethora of options for content of evaluation. Within the realm of professional psychology training, competency benchmarks (Hatcher et al., 2013) and evaluation methods (Kaslow et al., 2009) have been defined in a number of specialty areas. Competency-based models exist for psychologists specializing in primary care (APA, 2014; McDaniel et al., 2014), geropsychology (APA, 2014; Knight et al., 2009), health psychology (Larkin & Klonoff, 2014), and rehabilitation psychology (Stiers et al., 2012), as well as those working in interdisciplinary, integrated teams (e.g., APA, 2008) and rural settings (Riding-Malon & Werth, Jr., 2014). The field of social work also follows a competency-based model of training. Pertinent models for review, practice standards, and guidelines for social work practice are readily available from the National Association of Social Work (www.socialworkers.org/Practice/Practice-Standards-Guidelines). The American Association for Geriatric Psychiatry (www.aagponline. org) and the American Board of Psychiatry and Neurology (www.abpn. com) also list competency benchmarks and training requirements for specialization in geriatric psychiatry.

Training pre-licensed individuals to do home care is a very rewarding experience for both trainees and supervisors. Though home-care-based medical programs are becoming more available, this specialized training is not always offered in clinical training programs. Therefore, it is equally important for newly licensed MH professionals to seek ongoing training and professional development to provide effective MH services in the home setting.

Training Newly Licensed Mental Health Professionals

Home-based MH care practice demands a wide range of knowledge and skills in managing the MH needs of older adults, working as part of an interdisciplinary team, and providing care in the home setting (Hicken & Plowhead, 2010). Even newly licensed MH professionals who work in home care teams may not have received formal training and/or experience in integrated care, home care, and/or specialty training working with older adults. As such, they may need professional development resources and support to translate existing competencies and develop new ones to optimize quality practice in the home care setting'(Terry, Gordon, Steadman-Wood, & Karel, 2017).

Dr. Park received his doctorate in clinical psychology with a focus on geropsychology through his graduate studies, predoctoral internship, and postdoctoral fellowship. Upon completing his postdoctoral fellowship training, Dr. Park accepted a staff psychologist position in a VA HBPC program that provides integrated primary care and MH services to older adults. Dr. Park felt well suited to work with older Veterans, given his training in geropsychology, but had no experience providing home care services.

Dr. Park learned about the national VA HBPC MH provider community of practice. This community of practice has established numerous resources for professional development in HBPC which include: (1) a list-serve for communication, (2) an online internal repository that houses resources to orient and support newly hired HBPC MH providers, (3) a monthly educational webinar series, (4) ongoing performance improvement workgroups, and (5) an HBPC MH provider mentorship program where seasoned and newly hired HBPC MH providers are paired and engage in a mentorship relationship defined by the mentor and mentee. Dr. Park joined the list-serve, gained access to shared community resources, attended monthly webinars, and participated in the VA HBPC MH provider mentorship program to enhance his professional development.

After several years working as a VA HBPC staff psychologist, Dr. Park decided to pursue specialty certification in geropsychology, through the American Board of Professional Psychology (ABPP). Next, Dr. Park worked with the leaders of his local VA MH service and affiliated academic institution to develop a geropsychology internship and postdoctoral fellowship training program in HBPC.

As noted with Dr. Park's experience, the VA is a pioneer in HBPC MH service delivery. It has well-established programming to provide training and education to HBPC MH providers, including a series of self-study web courses describing a model of integrated MH assessment and treatment in VA HBPC. Several HBPC MH providers have made contributions to the literature specific to their work in this area; see, for example, Hicken and Plowhead (2010) on the nuances of psychological practice in HBPC, Terry and colleagues (2017) on the VA HBPC MH Provider Peer Mentorship Program, and Feng and colleagues (2017) on independent living capacity assessment in HBPC. In 2013, VA leadership published a paper on the national integration of MH providers in VA HBPC, demonstrating the effectiveness of this innovative model of home-based geriatric MH care (Karlin & Karel, 2014). Reckrey and colleagues have published several articles on community-based HBPC, including one (Reckrey et al., 2014) on the critical role of social workers on these teams. This paper includes a comprehensive history about demonstration projects to incentivize providers to provide cost-effective home care for medically frail, medically complex older adults.

Professional development opportunities can also be obtained through continuing education, specialty competency and board certification training, professional connections, consultation, and mentorship. Professional organizations (e.g., APA, American Psychiatric Association, National Association of Social Workers, Clinical Social Work Association, Home Centered Care Institute, and the Aging Life Care Association – formerly the National Association of Professional Geriatric Care Managers) offer a variety of continuing education resources related to integrated care, geriatrics, and home-based practice.

Dr. Sanchez, a newly licensed clinical psychologist, decided to relocate to be close to her family upon completing her training. Dr. Sanchez accepted a position as a staff psychologist in a family medicine practice working in an integrated, primary care behavioral health program. Over time, she realized that many of the older adult patients had difficulty coming to the clinic for their appointments, and when they did come in, their medical conditions were not optimally controlled. Dr. Sanchez approached the clinic medical director about the prospect of offering home-based integrated primary care behavioral health services. The medical director was supportive of the idea, and as part of the service delivery expansion plan, both Dr. Sanchez and the medical director sought additional professional training from the Home Centered Care Institute, a national, non-profit organization that educates, trains, and provides mentorship to clinicians and healthcare leaders to become successful HBPC providers. As the program expanded, Dr. Sanchez and her home care team implemented several quality improvement projects to objectively measure the impact of the improved access to care.

Licensed MH professionals require ongoing continuing education to maintain licensure and stay current in their respective fields, yet competency standards and practice guidelines for home-based MH providers are not well established (Hicken & Plowhead, 2010). The APA has published guidelines on working with older adults (APA, 2014) and in primary care psychology (APA, 2015), which are informative to psychologists providing home care. The ABPP offers specialty certification in the fields of geropsychology, health psychology, rehabilitation psychology, and neuropsychology that may be sought by psychologists providing MH services in the home setting. Professional organizations associated with other MH professions such as the National Association of Social Workers and the American Psychiatric Association offer communities of practice for continuing education, resource sharing, and communication that can be applied to working with older adults in home care setting. The vignettes above illustrate the variety of ways MH providers can seek additional training and ongoing training specific to home care.

Summary

Integrated home care is part of a growing movement in the United States to improve access to MH treatment (Choi, 2009), and therefore it is important to continue to build these communities of practice, establish competency standards, and provide training and ongoing professional development to prepare the home-based MH workforce to meet the demand.

Providing mental health services at home creates several unique opportunities and challenges that are not routinely encountered in more traditional MH care settings (Blass et al., 2006). Therefore, it is important that MH providers are aware of these potential issues to work effectively in the home care setting (Hicken & Plowhead, 2010). Training and ongoing professional development are ways in which MH providers hone and refine the skills to do this meaningful work.

Note

* It is critical that trainees be provided with clear instructions for when to call 911 for medical and/or psychiatric emergencies. Though relatively rare, crises do arise in the home care setting. A trainee may be the first person the patient comes into contact with during the day, and knowing what to do can be the difference between life and death. Always encourage trainees to consult with the supervisor and/or medical provider when needed. Reviewing policies and procedures often can also reduce the trainee's anxiety and improve the ability to act if a crisis should occur.

References

American Psychological Association (APA). (2008). *Blueprint for change: Achieving integrated health care for an aging population.* Retrieved from www.apa.org/pi/aging/programs/integrated/integrated-healthcare-report.pdf.

American Psychological Association (APA). (2014). Guidelines for psychological practice with older adults. *American Psychologist, 34*–65. doi:10.1037/a0035063.

American Psychological Association. (2015). *Competencies for Psychology Practice in Primary Care.* Retrieved from www.apa.org/ed/resources/competencies-practice.pdf.

American Psychological Association (APA). (2015). *Competencies for psychological practice with older adults.* Retrieved from www.apa.org/ed/resources/competencies-practice.pdf.

Blass, D. M., Rye, R. M., Robbins, B. M., Miner, M. M., Handel, S., Carroll, J. L., & Rabins, P. V. (2006). Ethical issues in mobile psychiatric treatment with homebound elderly patients: The Psychogeriatric Assessment and Treatment in City Housing experience. *Journal of the American Geriatrics Society, 54*, 843–848. doi:10.1111/j.1532-5415.2006.00706.

Choi, N. G. (2009). The integration of social and psychologic services to improve low-income homebound older adults' access to depression treatment. *Family & Community Health, 32*, S27–S35. doi:10.1097/01.FCH.0000342837.97982.36.

Feng, M. C., Murphy, M. R., & Mlinac, M. (2017). Independent living capacity evaluation in home-based primary care: Considerations and outcomes of quality improvement project. *Clinical Gerontologist, 40*, 51–62. doi:10.1080/07317115.2016.1210272.

Hatcher, R. L., Fouad, N. A., Grus, C. L., Campbell, L. F., McCutcheon, S. R., & Leahy, K. L. (2013). Competency benchmarks: Practical steps toward a culture of competence. *Training and Education in Professional Psychology, 7*, 84–91. doi:10.1037/a0029401.

Hicken, B. L., & Plowhead, A. (2010). A model for home-based psychology from the Veterans Health Administration. *Professional Psychology: Research and Practice, 41*, 340–346. doi:10.1037/a0020431.

Hinshaw, A. S. (1995). Toward achieving multidisciplinary professional collaboration. *Professional Psychology: Research and Practice, 26*, 115–116. doi:10.1037/0735-7028.26.2.115.

Karlin, B., & Karel, M. J. (2014). National integration of mental health providers in VA home-based primary care: A innovative model for mental health care delivery with older. *The Gerontologist, 54*, 1–12. doi:10.1093/geront/gnt142.

Kaslow, N. J., Grus, C. L., Campbell, L. F., Fouad, N. A., Hatcher, R. L., & Rodolfa, E. R. (2009). Competency assessment toolkit for professional psychology. *Training and Education in Professional Psychology, 3*, S27–S45. doi:10.1037/a0015833.

Knight, B. G., Karel, M. J., Hinrichsen, G. A., Qualls, S. H., & Duffy, M. (2009). Pikes Peak model for training in professional geropsychology. *American Psychologist, 6*, 205–214. doi:10.1037/a0015059.

Larkin, K. T., & Klonoff, E. A. (2014). *Specialty competencies in clinical health psychology*. New York: Oxford University Press.

McDaniel, S. H., Grus, C. L., Cubic, B. A., Hunter, C. L., Kearney, L. K., Schuman, C. C., … Bennett Johnson, S. (2014). Competencies for psychology practice in primary care. *American Psychologist, 69*, 409–429. doi:10.1037/a0036072.

Reckrey, J. M., Gettenberg, G. G., Ross, H., Kopke, V., Soriano, T., & Ornstein, K. (2014). The critical role of social workers in home-based primary care. *Social Work Health Care, 53*, 330–343. doi:10.1080/00981389.2014.884041.

Riding-Malon, R., & Werth, Jr., J. L. (2014). Psychological practice in rural settings: At the cutting edge. *Professional Psychology: Research and Practice, 45*, 85–91. doi:10.1037/a0036172.

Stiers, W., Barisa, M., Stucky, K., Barisa, M., Brownsberger, M., Van Tubbergen, M., … Kummel, A. (2012). Guidelines for competency development and measurement in rehabilitation psychology postdoctoral training. *Rehabilitation Psychology, 57*, 267–279. doi:10.1037/a0030774.

Terry, D. L., Gordon, H. B., Steadman-Wood, P., & Karel, M. J. (2017). A peer mentorship program for mental health professionals in Veterans Health Administration Home-Based Primary Care. *Clinical Gerontologist, 40*, 97–105. doi:10.1080/07317115.2016.1255691.

Yang, J. A., Garis, J., Jackson, C., & McClure, R. (2009). Providing psychotherapy to older adults in home: Benefits, challenges, and decision-making guidelines. *Clinical Gerontologist, 32*, 333–346. doi:10.1080/07317110902896356.

15 Special Considerations in Home Care

*Luis Richter, Ami Bryant, William Gibson,
and Clair Rummel*

This chapter will focus on other important considerations for home care mental health providers. Although each section could certainly be discussed within its own chapter, we would like to offer at least a primer for the following: suicide prevention, medical non-adherence, EOL care, and telehealth care. If a mental health (MH) provider would like to acquire further proficiency in one of these areas, additional resources will be discussed within each section.

Suicide Assessment and Prevention in Home Care

> During your initial assessment of a 77-year-old man recently discharged from the hospital, you notice that he has a significant amount of narcotic medications that have expired. In addition, he shares that he has not been sleeping well and that he feels a sense of purposelessness. You ask him about the surplus of medications and he says, "I am keeping them just in case I need a way out of this."

The need for suicide prevention in home care cannot be understated. Most patients enrolled in home care are older and have multiple chronic illnesses. Research has consistently found that suicide rates are higher among older adults as compared to other age groups (World Health Organization, 2014) and higher among patients with chronic illnesses (Fassberg et al., 2016). Among older adults, suicide attempts are more likely to be fatal. The rate of completed suicides to attempts is 1:4 among older adults compared to 1:100–200 for adults of all ages (Drapeau & McIntosh, 2016; Van Orden & Conwell, 2016). Older adults are also less likely to report suicidal thoughts as compared to younger adults (Duberstein et al., 1999). However, there are qualities of home care that enable the identification of suicide risk, and consequently lead to powerful preventative interventions.

First, home-based MH providers often work collaboratively as part of an interdisciplinary team. This increases the chance of identifying patients at risk for suicide (Van Orden & Conwell, 2016). MH providers can train team members to recognize warning signs for suicide and respond appropriately. If the MH provider does not work as part of an interdisciplinary team, collaboration with the patient's other providers is strongly encouraged.

Second, home care work poses unique safety concerns as the environment is not controlled in the manner of a typical clinical setting. If there is an immediate threat of danger either to the patient or the MH provider, emergency services should be called. If the MH provider feels it is safe, they should stay with the patient until emergency services arrive. However, if the MH provider deems it unsafe to remain in the situation, they should leave immediately and call emergency services.

Depending on the operating procedures of their agency, suicide screenings may be conducted by home care providers other than MH provider. At a minimum, suicidal ideation should be screened for during initial evaluations and at any point in treatment when warning signs are observed. Use of structured instruments to assist with screening are recommended (Corson, Gerrity, & Dobscha, 2004). Consider using one of the following:

• Beck Scale for Suicidal Ideation (BSS; Beck, Steer, & Ranieri, 1988).
• Beck Hopelessness Scale (BHS; Beck & Steer, 1988).
• Reasons for Living Inventory (RFL; Linehan et al., 1983).
• Columbia-Suicide Severity Rating Scale (C-SSRS; Posner et al., 2011).

Assessments specific to evaluating suicide in older adults may also be used:

• The Geriatric Suicide Ideation Scale (GSIS; Heisel & Flett, 2006).
• Reasons for Living Inventory-Older Adults (RFL-OA; Edelstein et al., 2009).

MH providers should carry materials needed for suicide risk screening, clinical risk assessments, and safety planning with them while in the field, as it is not always known when these materials will be needed.

If a patient screens positive for suicidal ideation, a clinical risk assessment is warranted (Wortzel, Matarazzo, & Homaifar, 2013). While an in-depth review of clinical suicide risk assessment is beyond the scope of this chapter, the following should be evaluated in a clinical suicide risk assessment:

1   Suicidal ideation (onset, frequency, duration, severity), intent, plan.
2   Access to means.
3   Warning signs.
4   Risk factors.
5   Protective factors.

Unstructured clinical interviews may fail to identify important information; thus, it is recommended that clinical risk assessments are conducted using structured instruments (Wortzel, Matarazzo, & Homaifar, 2013). The self-report instruments listed above are not only useful for screening but provide additional information that is useful for the clinical risk assessment.

Cognitive deficits may represent an additional challenge in suicide assessment (Van Orden & Conwell, 2016). If the patient has cognitive impairment or is an unreliable historian, the MH provider may find it helpful to obtain collateral information, assuming the patient provides permission. Relatives and other caregivers may have useful information regarding the patient's behaviors, recent emotional state, or expressions of distress.

After a clinical risk assessment has been completed, suicide risk should be stratified in terms of severity and temporality (Wortzel, Matarazzo, & Homaifar, 2013). An in-depth explanation of factors to consider when determining suicide risk can be found in the Therapeutic Risk Management Risk Stratification Tables available from the Rocky Mountain Mental Illness Research, Education, and Clinical Center: www.mirecc.va.gov/visn19/trm/ (MIRECC, n.d.) and in (Wortzel et al., 2014). After the risk level has been stratified, the appropriate level of care should be identified.

Following the clinical risk assessment, if emergency services are not warranted, a safety plan should be developed (Wortzel, Matarazzo, & Homaifar, 2013; Matarazzo, Homaifar, & Wortzel, 2014). See Conti and colleagues (2016) for a thorough explanation of how to collaboratively safety-plan with older adults. Within the context of home care, reducing access to lethal means is crucial (i.e. reducing access to firearms, stockpiled medications, etc.). Family members and caregivers can also assist with recognizing warning signs and in reducing access to lethal means, and provide coaching to the patient in use of their safety plan. If feasible, it can be efficient to have the patient fill out their own copy (or multiples) and find a suitable place to keep it (e.g., in the wallet, on the refrigerator). The safety plan should be reviewed and updated on a regular basis.

MH providers are likely to vary in terms of what suicide risk level they can effectively manage, based on a variety of factors such as agency regulations, caseload, etc. If the MH provider works as part of an interdisciplinary team, they can collaborate with team members on providing ongoing monitoring and interventions. Joint visits with team members may also be a helpful intervention. For example, if the patient receives visits from a recreation therapist for pleasant activities or receives exercise as part of visits from physical therapy, these pleasant and/or meaningful activities may be useful when developing interventions for the patient.

A variety of intervention strategies can be helpful for working with suicidal home care patients, including treating depression, enhancing coping skills, providing referrals for psychopharmacology if needed, and ensuring that the patient is aware of crisis resources. Increasing engagement in meaningful/pleasant activities, encouraging increased social contact, and reinforcing reasons for living may be especially important with the home care patient population. If the patient maintains the level of cognitive functioning necessary for cognitive restructuring, cognitive-based interventions to reframe and restructure suicidal thoughts may be helpful. If the patient has significant cognitive impairment, more concrete behavioral strategies may be more appropriate. In such cases, utilizing a family member or caregiver as a coach to reinforce behavioral strategies may help. Timely and effective EOL care is also a very powerful suicide-prevention intervention (this will be covered further in the EOL section below).

Medical Non-adherence

Ms. Jenkins refuses to take her medications despite numerous providers reminding her how important it is for her to do so. The home care team asks the MH provider, "Can you help us?"

Non-adherence issues in home care are common. MH providers are often tasked with consultation regarding the factors that may be contributing to this behavior, as well as recommendations on how to change the home care team's approach. When assessing the patient with non-adherence issues, such as medication non-adherence, several factors must be considered (see Table 15.1).

One of the most powerful contributions of an MH provider is helping to align the patient's values with the interventions and language used by the medical team. Often medical teams make well-intentioned recommendations and target critical medical outcomes that fail to be effective, simply because of the disconnect with the patient's own values and goals. Once the MH provider has helped patients articulate their own values and goals, the team might change the intervention, reframing their medical recommendations to match the patients' values and goals, or both.

Table 15.1 Assessment of Non-Adherence

Factors	Assessment Strategy
Cognitive impairment	Consider administering a cognitive screener or neuropsychological testing
Motivational factors	"On a scale of 1 to 10, how important is this change for you?" "On a scale of 1 to 10, how ready are you to change?" "On a scale of 1 to 10, how confident are you in changing this behavior?"
Logistical and financial barriers	Consider cost, transportation, access to food, access to care when applicable
Co-morbid MH diagnoses	Screen for mood, anxiety, personality disorders, and/or eating disorders when applicable
Caregiver and family issues	Explore whether family can support the patient in following the team's recommendation or do they represent a barrier or challenge? Is there caregiver burnout?
Sensory and functional limitations	Consider vision and hearing impairments, refer to physical or occupational therapy to consider physical limitations (e.g., finger dexterity for retrieving meds from pillbox)
Health literacy and family/cultural beliefs	Explore the patient's and the family/caregiver's level of health literacy. Explore family/cultural beliefs about health and medical care

An Example of Reframing

Home care team's goal: Improve patient's adherence to using walker to reduce the risk of falls. The team's insistence on the patient using the walker for *safety* does not convince the patient to use it. Why? Because you discover that the patient's goal is to maintain her independence and avoid appearing old among her peers. The patient states, "I do not want to use a walker – that makes me look old!" and "I am still independent, I do not need that."

Reframing the team's recommendation:

When you use your walker, you walk a lot faster and sturdier, you may even look younger. We know that maintaining your independence is really important to you, we want to support you with this. The best chance you have of maintaining independence is avoiding a fall, the walker will help you continue to live independently for as long as possible.

An Example of Expanding the Targets of Intervention and Reframing

Home care team's goal: Improve the patient's adherence to checking blood sugars daily and taking insulin as prescribed. The team's insistence on the patient adhering to the diabetes regimen to prevent further medical complications does not seem to compel the patient. His worst adherence is on weekends. Why? Because you discover that the patient's goal is to enjoy life without having to interrupt his favorite activities to check blood sugars or to take his insulin. His favorite activities include going on outings with his children every weekend, playing the piano, and watching baseball on television while texting his buddies who may also be watching the same game. The patient also states, "My health has been getting worse for years, I just want to enjoy as much as I can before it is time to check out" and "Checking my blood sugars gets in the way of what I love to do."

Reframing the team's recommendation:

> The risks of poorly controlled blood sugars may include neuropathy in your hands, this will make it difficult to play the piano or text your friends. The risks also include damage to your eyes, which will make it difficult for you to enjoy watching baseball on television. We know that enjoying activities with your grandchildren is important to you, and keeping your blood sugars well controlled will give you the best chance of continuing to do this as long as possible.

Expanding the targets of intervention: "Would it be okay if we include your children in conversations about your medical care, such as your blood sugars?"

When the MH provider is tasked to work directly with the patient on improving medical adherence, we would recommend a strong proficiency in motivational interviewing. For more information on acquiring motivational interviewing skills consider reading *Motivational Interviewing in Healthcare* by Rollnick and colleagues (2008), and/or *Motivational Interviewing for Clinical Practice* by Levounis and colleagues (2017), and enrolling in *in vivo* skills training by connecting with a certified trainer or workshop.

Weight Management and Pain Management

Non-adherence issues related to weight management and pain management are two very common reasons why an MH provider may be consulted, and these areas warrant their own discussion. However, we will not be able to explore these two complex areas with sufficient detail in this book. For MH providers interested in gaining further knowledge and expertise in these two areas, we do offer some reading recommendations. MH providers would benefit from becoming well versed in the "intuitive eating" arsenal of interventions, which represents a major empirically-based paradigm shift in weight management. Thus, we would recommend *Intuitive Eating* by Tribole and Resch (2012). For a comprehensive review of behavioral interventions for chronic pain, we recommend *Handbook of Psychosocial Intervention for Chronic Pain* (Maikovich-Fong, 2019).

End-of-Life Care

You have been asked to see Mr. Davis, a divorced Korean War veteran in his eighties with end-stage chronic obstructive pulmonary disease, who lives alone in a small apartment. He has some contact with some of his adult children but is estranged from others. This is partly due to the fact that, though he has been sober for many years, he developed a serious alcohol problem when he came back from Korea. His illness is terminal, and he is experiencing distress.

First, he feels very guilty about being estranged from some of his children. He would like to reconnect with them and make amends before he dies. Second, he feels he squandered many life opportunities because of his alcohol use. He is an intelligent man, but was never able to go to college because he had to work to support his family and drank heavily when he wasn't working. He wonders what he might have been able to accomplish had he been able to obtain sobriety sooner.

While Mr. Davis denies specific fear of death, he has begun to question his spiritual orientation. He was raised in a very strict fundamentalist church whose theology he found frightening, and stopped attending church as soon as he left home to join the Army. He doesn't believe in God in any traditional way but considers himself to be agnostic. As he nears death, he has begun to wonder about such things as the afterlife and the possibility of reincarnation.

Unlike colleagues in most other clinical settings, MH providers will often be called upon to work with people who are dying, and will do so in a wide variety of circumstances. In some cases, the patient will be an older person who has come to the end of his or her life naturally and will die a relatively peaceful death at home, surrounded by loving family. Many will be older adults who, like Mr. Davis, are dying from chronic, progressive illnesses such as pulmonary, renal, or cardiovascular disease. Others may have cancer or a dementing illness such as Alzheimer's, vascular, or Lewy body dementia. Some patients, particularly veterans, may be dealing with post-traumatic stress disorder (PTSD) or moral injury which they may never have addressed. Some may have been dealing with progressive decline for many years, while others will be newly diagnosed and/or will be experiencing a more rapid and/or unexpected decline. Each of these scenarios requires a somewhat different kind of response from MH providers; however, general principles and good psychological care and practice, with some modifications, apply to all EOL situations.

It is important to note that certain medical systems may contract outside agencies (with various compositions of interdisciplinary staff) to provide hospice services, whereas other systems offer this service within the scope of their own home care primary care team(s) and/or as an added specialty care service. Regardless, it is the MH provider's responsibility to understand the various disciplinary role and service differentiations within their particular medical system in order to provide and/or help shape the most effective collaboration for EOL care.

Block (2006) has suggested that "[p]sychological suffering is a virtually universal experience for patients at the end of life and for their families" (p. 751) and lists "[f]eelings of grief, sadness, despair, fear, anxiety, loss and loneliness" as common in patients who are facing death (p. 752).

General principles of therapeutic care apply at the end of life just as much as they do in any other therapeutic situation, if not more so. Abundant research supports the crucial role of forming a trusting therapeutic relationship, creating an expectation of benefit, and approaching patients with empathy, respect, and compassion (cf. Frank & Frank, 1993; Laska, Gurman, & Wampold, 2014; Wampold, 2012, 2015).

It is important to remember in this context that most people are very uncomfortable with death and don't know how to talk to those who are dying. As a result, the dying person often feels cut off from others and estranged from sources of support. Family and friends may stop coming to visit completely, or may visit but only be able to stay for short periods of time and talk only about superficial things, because of their own anxiety. Given this common scenario, it is critical that MH providers maintain the capacity to remain present and empathetic, explore deep and often fearful topics, and be willing, as much as possible, to follow their patients wherever they need to go in dealing with ultimate issues.

MH providers should familiarize themselves with the medical and psychological aspects of the diseases from which their patients are suffering, typical and pathological trajectories of loss and bereavement, and the psychological, sociocultural, spiritual, and interpersonal factors in chronic, advanced, life-limiting, and terminal illness (Kasl-Godley, King, & Quill, 2014). Included in this list is an assessment of the developmental issues the dying person may be facing – someone who is dying of ALS (amyotrophic lateral sclerosis) in her forties may be dealing with different challenges than a man who is dying of end-stage kidney disease in his eighties. Block (2006) suggests two useful questions to ask our dying patients to help begin the discussion:

> What is it like to be at this point in your life [finishing college, with young children, facing retirement, having lost your spouse] and facing a serious illness? What do you feel is the toughest loss for you at this stage in your life?
>
> (p. 753)

Finally, researchers (Kasl-Godley, King, & Quill, 2014; King & Wynne, 2004) emphasize the importance of also paying attention to family dynamics and developmental stage at the end of life. This is particularly salient for the MH providers who may have much more intimate contact with the terminally ill patient's family than providers working in more traditional clinical or hospital settings.

Grassman (2009) has articulated a set of five important tasks at the end of life, the completion of which may allow the patient and his or her family to navigate the dying process in a better, healthier fashion:

- Saying "thank you."
- Saying "I love you."
- Saying "I forgive you."
- Asking "Will you forgive me?"
- Saying "Goodbye."

Each person will think about and address these tasks in very different ways depending upon age, type of illness, speed of decline, and other factors. Whatever the specifics, these tasks can form a general framework the MH provider can use to help his or her patient explore interpersonal relationships at the end of life. This may involve working with the patient's family, friends, co-workers, those with whom they've been in conflict, and even pets. Grassman also highlights the importance of symbol and ritual in helping the dying person address these tasks and, one hopes, reaching a place of greater peace with death.

Research suggests that spirituality may serve as an important protective factor to depression and despair at the end of life (McClain, Rosenfeld, & Breitbart, 2003). Addressing spirituality and meaning with those who are dying is an important and often neglected area in psychological care of the dying (cf. Rego & Nunes, 2019; Rego et al., 2018). Having at least a basic familiarity with different religious and spiritual belief systems and comfort in being able to talk to patients in those terms is invaluable for the MH provider working with those who are dying. Consultation with the Chaplain Service and/or community clergy can aid in this process.

Aside from addressing specific religious or spiritual issues with their patients, MH provider working with people at the end of life are frequently confronted with the need to help their patients address existential issues involving not only some of the themes noted above (relationships, spirituality), but also meaning, autonomy, guilt, choice, and death anxiety.

The MH provider has a choice of using an arsenal of different formulated approaches. Kasl-Godley, King, and Quill (2014) describe potential adaptations of motivational interviewing, life review, cognitive behavioral therapy, and acceptance and commitment therapy for use with those at the end of life. LeMay and Wilson (2008) reviewed a long list of treatments designed to address existential distress. Breitbart and colleagues (2004, 2010, 2012) developed an approach based on Viktor Frankl's logotherapy for use with those dying of cancer, but which can be adapted to other terminal illnesses. Dignity therapy is another approach, which has been specifically studied in home care settings (Chochinov et al., 2005, 2011). Dignity therapy is a flexible approach that explicitly invites patients to discuss the themes that matter most to them as they approach death and offers open-ended questions to facilitate discussion. Themes include generativity, continuity of self, role preservation, maintenance of pride, hopefulness, aftermath concerns, and "care tenor" (how others interact with and respond to them). Dignity therapy also explicitly encourages the person who is dying to share the results of these discussions with family and others who are important in their lives, thus opening up opportunities to address interpersonal issues.

Whatever approach one takes, it is important to remain flexible and willing to stray from a protocol in order to address your patients' needs based on their own values as they wrestle with issues of spirituality and meaning at the end of their lives.

David Kissane and his colleagues (Kissane, Clarke, & Street, 2001; Robinson et al., 2015) have identified a specific configuration of features that can add additional distress to the dying process and make care of the dying person more challenging. They termed this particular configuration – hopelessness, loss of meaning, and existential distress – "demoralization syndrome," and they and others (Grassi & Nanni, 2016; Ko et al., 2018; Mogos, Roffey, & Thangathurai, 2013) have demonstrated its potential correlation with greater distress, a greater sense of being a burden, an increased wish for death, and even a greater risk for suicide among various populations at the end of life. Demoralization syndrome is not the same as, and should be carefully distinguished from, depression. Once the psychologist has identified the presence of the elements of demoralization syndrome, he or she can use one or more of the approaches described above to address this painful state.

Finally, the MH provider may need to help patients address PTSD or moral injury at the end of life. Space does not permit a detailed discussion of this topic, but Block (2006), Feldman and Periyakoil (2006), and Grassman (2009) all offer useful insights into addressing PTSD at the end of life. To date, there is no literature on addressing moral injury at the end of life, but see Litz et al. (2015), Lettini and Brock (2012), and Shay (1994) for general discussion about moral injury and potential ways to address it.

All who care for those at EOL need to be very mindful of their own attitudes towards death and dying. While we all know in the abstract that we will die, facing the deaths of others on a regular basis forces us more than most to confront the realities of death and the uncertainties surrounding its manner and timing. As much as possible, we need to develop healthy attitudes that can help us maintain a compassionate presence for our patients while also maintaining good boundaries. The latter is particularly challenging, since there are few more intimate tasks than caring for the dying, especially in a home setting. If the MH provider finds he or she is uncomfortable or feels out of his or her depth in addressing a particular topic or area, as always consultation, peer supervision, and/or supervision with a senior colleague can help the MH provider through these rough periods. Especially when dealing with such deep and fearful issues, there is no shame in leaning on colleagues for education and support. As we noted above in dealing with the tasks of dying, symbol and ritual can also be very helpful for teams of providers who deal with the death of patients on a regular basis. For example, conducting some kind of memorial monthly, quarterly, or annually, or even having a moment of silence or reading the names of the patients who have died, can help the team process their grief.

Many people presume that working with patients at the end of life is depressing. Quite the contrary; it can be among the most rewarding and useful work an MH provider can do.

Telemental Health

> Mrs. Kelsko, an 83-year-old widow, lives alone in rural Montana – three hours from the nearest medical center. She is depressed about losing her ability to ride horses and she can no longer drive, but she is adamant about continuing to live in her home for as long as possible. Family visit her often, but home care options are limited.

Numerous barriers to MH treatment exist for older adults, including geographic isolation, transportation limitations, stigma concerns, access to specialty providers, and mobility issues (Egede et al., 2015; Gentry, Lapid, & Rummans, 2019). Telemental health offers an effective approach to address these barriers and increase access to MH care. Telemental health can also decrease patient costs due to lower need for transportation resources, less missed work for caregivers, and enhanced provider productivity over standard outpatient or home-based care (Egede et al., 2015). For the purposes of this chapter, *telemental health* refers to MH services provided by a licensed MH provider via real-time videoconferencing transmitted via the internet (Turvey et al., 2013). Telemental health can be used as a supplement to home care or as a stand-alone modality.

Telemental health was initially delivered from clinic to clinic, in which the patient traveled to a local clinic and connected via videoconferencing to a provider located at another clinic. In the past several years, providers have begun to expand services to provide telemental health care directly into a patient's home. This direct-to-patient provision of care has further reduced the barriers to evidence-based care for older adults.

Telemental health for older adults is feasible and well accepted in the areas of nursing home consultation, cognitive testing, dementia care, and psychotherapy (Gentry, Lapid, & Rummans, 2019). Telemental health has been shown to be as effective as same-room care for older adults with depression treated via problem-solving therapy (Choi et al., 2014) or behavioral activation (Egede et al., 2015). Recent studies found that older adults are interested in this novel approach to care and there are no significant differences in the areas of service delivery perception, treatment credibility, and satisfaction when compared with same-room care (Egede et al., 2016; Greenwald et al., 2018).

In the following paragraphs we will review current best practices and provide real-world recommendations on how to most effectively treat older adults via telehealth. For a full review of telemental health best practices, including technical considerations, see the recent guidelines developed by the American Psychiatric Association and the American Telemedicine Association (Shore et al., 2018).

Administrative Considerations

Qualifications and Licensing

Providers of telemental health services must practice due diligence to ensure they follow state licensure laws in both the state in which they are practicing as well as the state where the patient is receiving care. If they are providing services within a federal healthcare system, then they must follow the specific organizational guidelines around licensure. These requirements can vary and are evolving, so providers should remain abreast of changes.

Scope of Practice

Providers should provide the same standard of care they provide in same-room care. In addition, multiple professional organizations have issued clinical practice guidelines for telehealth; for example, the American Psychological Association's 2013 Guidelines for Telepsychology. It is important for providers to be familiar with these and able to apply them when appropriate.

Procedures and Protocols

Providers should establish a set of standard operating procedures and protocols that cover a range of administrative and clinical issues. Of primary importance is a clear protocol for emergency situations. If the patient is receiving telemental health services at a clinic, the emergency protocol should be coordinated with on-site staff. For services provided directly to the patient's home, review of the emergency protocol should explicitly occur during the initial session.

Prior to initiating each session, and once the patient can confirm they are in a private area to preserve confidentiality, the following information should be verified:

1   Name of the patient.
2   Location of the patient during the session.
3   Current contact information for both the patient and the provider.
4   If services are provided to the patient's home, the name of an emergency contact.

It is of utmost importance to clarify the patient's location as the location may impact the emergency management protocol as well as licensure requirements, mandatory reporting, and related ethical requirements. In the case of non-cooperation from a patient and his/her support person, providers should be prepared to work with local emergency personnel to initiate emergency services or involuntary hospitalizations. It is important for providers to be familiar with local civil commitment regulations and to develop a relationship with local services to facilitate transfer of care, if needed.

Clinical Considerations

Assessing Appropriateness

Per recent guidelines, there is no research suggesting that telemental health is contraindicated for specific patient groups (Shore et al., 2018). However, there are individual factors to consider. For patients being seen at home, one must consider their ability to arrange for a private location, cooperate regarding safety issues, and effectively operate relevant technology. They must also have access to high-speed internet and the appropriate technology. Additional areas to consider include a patient's geographic distance to emergency services, the presence and abilities of the patient's support system, cognitive capacity, history of cooperation with MH treatment, current and past substance use, and history of violence or self-harm behaviors. These areas should be considered both at the point of agreeing to a referral and throughout treatment. During the consent process it is important to discuss that services may be discontinued or transferred to in-person care if the patient can no longer be safely managed via telehealth.

Informed Consent

Informed consent should occur at the start of services in compliance with state and federal laws. The consent process should include the same information reviewed during the same-room care as well as information specific to telemental health services. Important topics to review include the limits of confidentiality, the protocol in case of technical failure, guidelines for contact between sessions, conditions under which telemental health services may be terminated, and the emergency protocol.

Privacy and the Physical Environment

Providers of telemental health services must comply with all federal and state privacy requirements. Both the location of the provider and the patient are considered patient exam rooms. Providers should ensure that the session content cannot be overheard, and advise patients to conduct the session in a private setting. As best as possible, set the provider's and the patient's cameras at eye level. In setting up your telehealth workspace, light should be optimized (i.e. avoid back-lighting). Providers should be aware of what is visible to the patient, including the background, and set up the space to reflect a professional MH setting.

Practical Recommendations

Most evidence-based treatments can be implemented via telehealth without significant modification. One area to consider is how to provide your patient with relevant worksheets or written materials. Access to secure messaging via a patient portal is ideal. If that is not an option, materials can be mailed. It can also be very helpful to utilize software that allows you to share your screen with your patient. This can be utilized to review self-report measures, demonstrate how to complete a worksheet, or collaboratively set an agenda.

It is also beneficial to discuss in-home telemental health guidelines during the initial session. Guidelines should include reminders to conduct sessions in a private location, limit distractions during the session, dress appropriately, refrain from smoking or using other substances during the session, and fully charge devices prior to the appointment. A thorough review of the guidelines can prevent therapy-interring issues from coming up later.

References

Beck, A. T., & Steer, R. A. (1988). *Manual for Beck Hopelessness Scale*. San Antonio, TX: Psychological Corporation.

Beck, A. T., Steer, R. A., & Ranieri, W. F. (1988). Scale for suicide ideation: Psychometric properties of a self-report version. *Journal of Clinical Psychology*, 44, 499–505.

Block, S. D. (2006). Psychological issues in end-of-life care. *Journal of Palliative Medicine*, 9, 751–772.

Breitbart, W., Gibson, C., Poppito, S., & Berg, A. (2004). Psychotherapeutic interventions at the end of life: A focus on meaning and spirituality. *Canadian Journal of Psychiatry*, 49, 366–372.

Breitbart, W., Poppito, S., Rosenfeld, B., Vickers, A. J., Li, Y., Abbey, J., ... & Cassileth, B. R. (2012). Pilot randomized controlled trial of individual meaning-centered psychotherapy for patients with advanced cancer. *Journal of Clinical Oncology*, 30, 1304–1309.

Breitbart, W., Rosenfeld, B., Gibson, C., Pessin, H., Poppito, S., Nelson, C., ... & Sorger, B. (2010). Meaning-centered group psychotherapy for patients with advanced cancer: A pilot randomized controlled trial. *Psycho-oncology*, 19, 21–28.

Chochinov, H. M., Hack, T., Hassard, T., Kristjanson, L. J., McClement, S., & Harlos, M. (2005). Dignity therapy: A novel therapeutic intervention for patients near the end of life. *Journal of Clinical Oncology*, 23, 5520–5525.

Chochinov, H. M., Kristjanson, L. J., Breitbart, W., McClement, S., Hack, T. F., Hassard, T., & Harlos, M. (2011). Effect of dignity therapy on distress and end-of-life experience in terminally ill patients: A randomised controlled trial. *The Lancet Oncology*, 12, 753–762.

Choi, N. G., Hegel, M. T., Marti, C. N., Marinucci, M. L., Sirrianni, L., & Bruce, M. L. (2014). Telehealth problem-solving therapy for depressed low-income homebound older adults. *The American Journal of Geriatric Psychiatry*, 22, 263–271. doi:10.1016/j.jagp.2013.01.037.

Conti, E. C., Arnspiger, B., Uriarte, J., Kraus-Schuman, C., & Batiste, M. (2016). *Collaborative safety planning for older adults*. Washington, DC: United States Department of Veterans Affairs. Retrieved from www.mirecc.va.gov/VISN16/docs/Safety_Planning_for_Older_Adults_Manual.pdf.

Corson, K., Gerrity, M. S., & Dobscha, S. K. (2004). Screening for depression and suicidality in a VA primary care setting: 2 items are better than 1 item. *The American Journal of Managed Care*, 10, 839–845.

Drapeau, C. W. & McIntosh, J.L. (2016). *U.S.A. suicide: 2015 official final data*. Washington, DC: American Association of Suicidology.

Duberstein, P. R., Conwell, Y., Sedlitz, L., Lyness, J. M., Cox, C., & Caine, E. D. (1999). Age and suicidal ideation in older depressed inpatients. *The American Journal of Geriatric Psychiatry, 7,* 289–296.

Edelstein, B. A., Heisel, M. J., Mckee, D. R., Martin, R. R., Koven, L. P., Duberstein, P. R., & Britton, P. C. (2009). Development and psychometric evaluation of the reasons for living–older adults scale: A suicide risk assessment inventory. *The Gerontologist, 49*(6), 736–745. doi:10.1093/geront/gnp052.

Egede, L. E., Acierno, R., Knapp, R. G., Lejuez, C., Hernandez-Tejada, M., Payne, E. H., & Frueh, B. C. (2015). Psychotherapy for depression in older veterans via telemedicine: A randomized, open-label, non-inferiority trial. *Lancet Psychiatry, 2,* 693–701. doi:10.1016/S2215-0366(15)00122-4.

Egede, L. E., Acierno, R., Knapp, R. G., Walker, R. J., Payne, E. H., & Frueh, B. C. (2016). Psychotherapy for depression in older veterans via telemedicine: Effect on quality of life, satisfaction, treatment credibility and service delivery perception. *Journal of Clinical Psychiatry, 77,* 1704–1711. doi:10.4088/JCP.16m10951.

Fassberg, M. M., Cheung, G., Canetto, S. S., Erlangsen, A., Lapierre, S., Linder, R., ... Waern, M. (2016). A systematic review of physical illness, functional disability, and suicidal behavior among older adults. *Aging & Mental Health, 20,* 166–194. doi:10.1080/13607863.2015.1083945.

Feldman, D. B., & Periyakoil, V. S. (2006). Posttraumatic stress disorder at the end of life. *Journal of Palliative Medicine, 8,* 213–218.

Frank, J. D., & Frank, J. B. (1993). *Persuasion and healing: A comparative study of psychotherapy.* Baltimore, MD: Johns Hopkins University Press.

Gentry, M. T., Lapid, M. I., & Rummans, T. A. (2019). Geriatric telepsychiatry: Systematic review and policy considerations. *The American Journal of Geriatric Psychiatry, 27,* 109–127. doi:10.1016/j.jagp.2018.10.009.

Grassi, L., & Nanni, M. G. (2016). Demoralization syndrome: New insights in psychosocial cancer care. *Cancer, 122,* 2130–2133.

Grassman, D. L. (2009). *Peace at last: Stories of hope and healing for veterans and their families.* St. Petersburg, FL: Vandamere Press.

Greenwald, P., Stern, M.E., Clark, S., & Sharma, R. (2018). Older adults and technology: in telehealth, they may not be who you think they are. *Int. J. Emerg. Med., 11*(1), 2.

Heisel, M. J., & Flett, G. L. (2006). The development and initial validation of the geriatric suicide ideation scale. *The American Journal of Geriatric Psychiatry, 14,* 742–751. doi:10.1097/01.jgp.0000218699.27899.f9.

Kasl-Godley, J. E., King, D. A., & Quill, T. E. (2014). Opportunities for psychologists in palliative care. *American Psychologist, 69,* 364–376.

King, D. A., & Wynne, L. C. (2004). The emergence of "family integrity" in later life. *Family Process, 43,* 7–21.

Kissane, D. W., Clarke, A. M., & Street, A. F. (2001). Demoralization syndrome – A relevant psychiatric diagnosis for palliative care. *Journal of Palliative Care, 17,* 12–21.

Ko, K.-T., Lin, C.-J., Pi, S.-H., Li, Y.-C., & Fang, C.-K. (2018). Demoralization syndrome among elderly patients with cancer disease. *International Journal of Gerontology, 12*(1), 12–16.

Laska, K. M., Gurman, A. S., & Wampold, B. E. (2014). Expanding the lens of evidence-based practice in psychotherapy: A common factors perspective. *Psychotherapy, 51,* 467–481.

LeMay, K., & Wilson, K. (2008). Treatment of existential distress in life-threatening illness: A review of manualized interventions. *Clinical Psychology Review, 28,* 472–493.

Lettini, G., & Brock, R. N. (2012). *Soul repair: Recovering from moral injury after war.* Boston, MA: Beacon Press.

Levounis, P., Baachar, A., & Marienfield, C. (2017). *Motivational interviewing for clinical practice.* Washington, DC: American Psychiatric Association Publishing.

Linehan, M. M., Goodstein, J. L., Nielsen, S. L., & Chiles, J. A. (1983). Reasons for staying alive when you are thinking of killing yourself: The reasons for living inventory. *Journal of Consulting and Clinical Psychology, 51,* 276–286. doi:10.1037/0022-006x.51.2.276.

Litz, B. T., Lebowitz, L., Gray, M. J., & Nash, W. P. (2015). *Adaptive disclosure: A new treatment for military trauma, loss, and moral injury.* New York, NY: Guilford Press.

Maikovich-Fong, A. K. (Ed). (2019). *Handbook of psychosocial interventions for chronic pain: An evidence-based guide.* New York, NY: Routledge.

Matarazzo, B. B., Homaifar, B. Y., & Wortzel, H. S. (2014). Therapeutic risk management of the suicidal patient: Safety planning. *Journal of Psychiatric Practice, 20,* 220–224.

McClain, C. S., Rosenfeld, B. D., & Breitbart, W. (2003). Effect of spiritual well-being on end-of-life despair in terminally-ill cancer patients. *The Lancet, 361,* 1603–1607.

Mogos, M., Roffey, P., & Thangathurai, D. (2013). Demoralization syndrome: A condition often undiagnosed in terminally ill patients. *Journal of Palliative Medicine, 16,* 601.

Posner, K., Brown, G. K., Stanley, B., Brent, D. A., Yershova, K. V., Oquendo, M. A., … Mann, J. J. (2011). The Columbia–Suicide Severity Rating Scale: Initial validity and internal consistency findings from three multisite studies with adolescents and adults. *American Journal of Psychiatry, 168,* 1266–1277. doi:10.1176/appi.ajp.2011.10111704.

Rego, F., & Nunes, R. I. (2019). The interface between psychology and spirituality in palliative care. *Journal of Health Psychology, 24,* 279–287.

Rego, F., Pereira, C., Rego, G., & Nunes, R. (2018). The psychological and spiritual dimensions of palliative care: A descriptive systematic review. *Neuropsychiatry, 8,* 484–494.

Robinson, S., Kissane, D. W., Brooker, J., & Burney, S. (2015). A systematic review of the demoralization syndrome in individuals with progressive disease and cancer: A decade of research. *Journal of Pain and Symptom Management, 49,* 595–610.

Rocky Mountain Mental Illness Research, Education and Clinical Center (MIRECC). (n.d.). Therapeutic risk management- Risk stratification table. Retrieved from www.mirecc.va.gov/visn19/trm/docs/RM_MIRECC_SuicideRisk_Table.pdf.

Rollnick, S., Miller, W. H., & Butler, C. (2008). *Motivational interviewing in healthcare: Helping patients change behavior.* New York, NY: Guilford Publications.

Shay, J. (1994). *Achilles in Vietnam: Combat trauma and the undoing of character.* New York, NY: Scribner.

Shore, J. H., Yellowless, P., Caudill, R., Johnston, B., Turvey, C., Mishkind, M., ... Hilty, D. (2018). Best practices in videoconferencing-based telemental health April 2018. *Telemedicine and e-Health, 24*, 827–832. doi:10.1089/tmj.2018.0237.

Tribole, E., & Resch, E. (2012). *Intuitive eating: A revolutionary program that works.* New York, NY: Guilford Press.

Turvey, C., Coleman, M., Dennison, O., Drude, K., Goldenson, M., Hirsch, P., ... Bernard, J. (2013). ATA practice guidelines for video-based online mental health services. *Telemedicine Journal and e-Health, 19*, 722–730. doi:10.1089/tmj.2013.9989.

Van Orden, K. A., & Conwell, Y. (2016). Issues in research on aging and suicide. *Aging & Mental Health, 20*, 240–251. doi:10.1080/13607863.2015.1065791.

Wampold, B. E. (2012). Humanism as a common factor in psychotherapy. *Psychotherapy, 49*, 444–449.

Wampold, B. E. (2015). How important are the common factors in psychotherapy? An update. *World Psychiatry, 14*, 270–277.

World Health Organization. (2014). *Prevention suicide: A global imperative.* Geneva: World Health Organization.

Wortzel, H. S., Homaifar, B., Matarazzo, B., & Brenner, L. A. (2014). Therapeutic risk management of the suicidal patient: Stratifying risk in terms of severity and temporality. *Journal of Psychiatric Practice, 20*, 63–77.

Wortzel, H. S., Matarazzo, B., & Homaifar, B. A. (2013). A model for therapeutic risk management of the suicidal patient. *Journal of Psychiatric Practice, 19*, 323–326.

Index

Page numbers in **bold** refer to tables.

Printed in the United States
By Bookmasters